Dare to Fly

A Surgeon's Story

Sat Mehta

Nettle Books

Published 2022 by Nettle Books, Yorkshire
nettlebooks4@gmail.com
Revised edition

©2022 Sat Mehta
ISBN: 978-0-9933729-9-5
Classification: Biography

Acknowledgements

I am indebted to my hero, Professor Robert Rauf, who inspired me to follow my dream, and become a surgeon. I am also indebted to my children and grandchildren who are a continual source of love, life and laughter.

The events and clinical scenarios chronicled in this book happened in real life, but names and other identifying features have been changed to protect the privacy of colleagues and patients.

Front cover picture: Kate Mehta

Dedication

To my five beautiful granddaughters
– Sara, Molly, Holly, Anya, and Hattie –
who now know that Grandpa was once
young.
And to my four wonderful children
– Louise, Paul, Clare and Jane –
who have allowed me to tell their story.
And finally to my wife Kate –
without your help, my books would not have
been written.

Contents

Prologue, 5
1: Passage to England, 11
2: Worcester Sauce, 19
3: Cambridge and Plymouth, 26
4: Robin Hood Country, 31
5: Doctor in Danger, 39
6: A Very English Romance, 45
7: Wedding Bells, 55
8: Lincolnshire, 62
9: A Spiritual Journey, 69
10: The Midlands, 77
11: Country Life, 82
12: Children, 85
13: Kate Goes to India, 99
14: White Rose County, 113
15: Friends, 118
16: Tales from Barnsley, 123
17: Unusual Cases, 132
18: The Visit, 137
19: Travels, 145
20: Kate's Dad Goes to India Too, 157
21: Generations, 172
22: Our Family and Other Pets, 177
23: Relatives, 186
24: Lull Before the Storm, 191
Epilogue, 201
Afterword, 204

Prologue

MONDAY NIGHT was badminton night. I played in the Wakefield League. My partner was my tall and elegant neighbour. We made a good team, as she played at the base line and I played at the net. We often played against youngsters half our age and the pace was fast and furious.

One night, after a league match, I had a pain in my chest and down my left arm, radiating to my fingers. It lasted a few seconds. When I arrived home, I mentioned the chest pain to my wife Kate, and we agreed it was indigestion. She slid a couple of antacid tablets over the kitchen table, and we thought no more about it.

The "indigestion" went on for two years and we treated it with the same simple remedy. Eventually Kate decided to find out if anything more serious was going on. She arranged for a gastric camera examination.

I sat in my colleague's clinic as he said: "Nothing there, Sat. Tell me your symptoms again," I repeated my symptoms and we both knew then, *exactly* what was wrong.

"Sat," he said gravely," I'm sending you to the Cardiac Department." I went on the treadmill whilst my heart was monitored, and there it was, that familiar pain – angina. Only the previous year I had run a half marathon and I am thankful that I did not drop-down dead!

An angiogram of the blood vessels surrounding my heart showed they were obstructed with plaque. Three of the four vessels supplying my heart muscle were severely narrowed and inaccessible to a cardiac catheter. I could not have an *angioplasty* – that is, a catheter threaded into the coronary arteries to insert spring-loaded stents to keep the arteries open.

I moved up to the next level. We knew this was a very serious situation. Finley Crawshaw, the Professor of Cardiac Surgery, had a pleasant waiting room, a large store-room where he kept patients' notes in about forty huge trolleys, and a small office. He said we had three options: do nothing, treat medically or treat surgically. The first two options would allow me to lead a slower pace of life with a variety of restrictions. The third option came with some serious risks.

The surgical procedure would be to cut through my sternum, move my ribs out of the way and replace the blocked arteries with a breast artery diverted from my chest wall and veins from my leg. The Professor outlined the risks of surgery. He said: "Two per cent die on the table, about four per cent die within the first ten days, and twenty per cent live five years. The remainder are alive and well twenty or thirty years hence."

He said we could think about it and to let him know whether we wished to start medication or go for surgery. Kate and I looked at each other and immediately we knew I could not live life as an invalid. We were willing to take the surgical risk, the sooner the better. "I thought so," he said, "I've got a slot next Monday if you want to take it."

It was a lot to take in. I was forty-eight years old. We went home and for the next week went through the motions of everyday living as if nothing life-changing was about to happen.

Two days before my admission to hospital, my sister-in-law phoned. She and her family had moved in with my father-in-law Tony some years before. "I'm bringing Dad over," she said, "He's got a terrible pain in his eye, so see what you can do for him." And she dropped him off with us.

6

I took Tony to see my colleague, the Ophthalmic Surgeon. He treated Tony's eye with Laser Surgery. My colleague was very unhappy that the symptoms of the Glaucoma from which Tony suffered had been neglected, and he was unable to save the sight in his left eye. "If you'd come to me sooner," he said, "I could have saved the sight in this eye." He admitted Tony to his ward for an overnight stay. Tony then stayed with us for six weeks before returning to the house in Lincolnshire which he shared with his youngest daughter and her husband.

When we collected him the following day, he had a dressing over his eye and a large quantity of eye drops in a Hospital Pharmacy paper bag. "You'll have to help me," he said, waving the bag, "because I can't see straight, "He added "I need these eye drops every *two hours!*"

I had cancelled my operating list and clinics and informed my colleagues I would be away for a few weeks following my operation. My friends and colleagues were bewildered why I should have developed this condition. I am small, underweight and active; and, as a friend said: "When did you *ever* eat a chip, Sat? If this has happened to you, what chance have the rest of us?"

In my case, the cause is genetic, accelerated by the cloud of anxiety I had worked under for the past four years, and the doubling of my workload. I had run Barnsley's ENT Department single-handed until the eventual appointment of another ENT Consultant only three months previously.

The day before my operation was a Sunday. I went to church and my friends there were amazed and very supportive. Immediately afterwards, I went to the hospital and surrendered myself to major surgery. The admission paperwork done, I was shaved once, and then once more, from the neck to the ankles, and dressed in a backless hospital gown. I was a chicken, plucked and dressed, ready for the pot.

The anaesthetist explained, in the most jovial terms, how I would be virtually frozen, my heartbeats would be stopped, and my blood diverted for re-oxygenation, to a machine beside the table. After the breast artery was freed for re-directing to my heart, a vein would be stripped from my leg, then both used to repair the blockages. I would then hopefully be re-connected, and my sternum wired together. Closed, padded up, and smelling strongly of anaesthetic gases, I would then be dispatched to the Intensive Coronary Care Unit.

Early next morning, I was taken to the operating theatre. I understand my triple bypass coronary operation took four hours. I spent three days in the Intensive Care ward, of which I remember nothing.

Kate was invited by the anaesthetist to be at my bedside when he reversed my heavy sedation, and I would regain consciousness. Around my bed was an audience of medical staff, all waiting to see me return to the real world. I was disconnected from the breathing ventilator, the reversal drug was given, and they stood back and awaited the miracle. Nothing happened.

Seconds went by, and Kate, hopping from one foot to another, grew anxious. The anaesthetist, a very experienced practitioner, had seen this many times and knew what to expect. He said, "Tell him to breathe, Mrs Mehta."

Kate leaned over and yelled: "BREATHE, SAT, BREATHE!" At which point I took an almighty breath and Kate beamed at us all. "You see," said the anaesthetist to the assembled crowd, "He just daren't do anything else. Even under anaesthesia, he does what she tells him!"

I improved enough to move to the main hospital ward. It suited me to be with other patients. I had chest drains, tubes, a drip, and two enormous wound dressings and took regular painkillers.

Kate found it hard going, with four young children, an elderly father requiring two-hourly eye drops and a very sick husband in hospital. She phoned both her sisters in Lincolnshire, but they could not help. She phoned a friend nearby, but *she* said: "Sorry, can't help I'm stocktaking."

Eventually Kate phoned Brian, her cousin, "I can't cope," she said simply. Brian was a police officer with Strathclyde Police Force. He had three young children and a very sick wife of his own, but he replied: "Leave it with me, Kathleen."

Four hours later he knocked on our door. He had driven 250 miles to stay with us and help in our darkest hour. Kate and Brian visited me every day and they looked after my father-in-law at home as well. Brian stayed a week and shared the burden of care, the grocery shopping, the cooking, and the driving back and forth to Sheffield to visit me, and took care of Tony's eye drops. He even made sure that Kate ate her meals and took enough rest.

Since then, Kate has adopted him as her Wonderful Brother. We will never forget his kindness in our hour of need.

During my stay in hospital, I noticed several patients who had similar procedures to mine and were very ill. There were also some heart transplant patients in the ward. One afternoon, as I was lying in my bed, I noticed that the patient opposite was having problems breathing and was getting very panicky. I tried to alert some nursing staff, but with no success; I saw he became very pale and stopped moving. I realised something was seriously wrong, so I took my drip stand, tubes and bags, and walked across, prepared to give cardiac massage. A nurse ran up the ward and took over.

I was reprimanded and put in a side ward near the nursing station. I was banned from moving from my bed; and when Kate and Brian visited later that day, the nurse said "Ah, Mr Mehta, we've put him in the side ward." She chuckled. "I'm afraid you'll find him a bit sleepy." They had me well sedated.

Five days later I was discharged home. The surgeon warned me I might suffer from a "frozen chest" for the foreseeable future, restricting my rib movement during breathing. I thought this was perfectly reasonable as I had been opened and my ribs spread out like a smoked fish.

I had physiotherapy at the hospital following the operation, but nothing was arranged for home. The following week I developed a chest infection because, as predicted, I could not expand my rib cage to breathe. Kate thought we should continue with further physiotherapy at home to improve breathing and help with the healing.

We invited our friend's daughter, a recently qualified physiotherapist, to teach Kate chest physiotherapy. She was very kind and came straight away. She showed chest expanding exercises and postural drainage technique: this requires the patient to lie with the upper chest hanging over the foot of the bed, face down, and head over a bowl, whilst a helper pummels the back to help loosen secretions that are then coughed up into the bowl.

Kate was amused to read in our young daughter Jane's school exercise book Jane's account of postural drainage. She began: "My Daddy has had a very big operation. But it's alright, he is back home again now. I can hear Mummy banging Daddy in the bedroom upstairs."

So, my operation had been a success, but my life had been changed forever.

1. Passage to England

I QUALIFIED with a Bachelor of Medicine and a Bachelor of Surgery degree from Amritsar Medical School, India, in the summer of 1964 . I took up my first job in the prestigious All India Institute of Medical Sciences in Delhi. Junior doctors moved jobs every six months in those days, to gain experience in every branch of their profession, so the next job I took was at Irwin Hospital, also in Delhi.

Readers of my first memoir *Flying with a Broken Wing* will know this was the same hospital in which I lay as a boy, fifteen years previously, waiting for my infected arm to be amputated above the elbow. But a miracle happened, and the arm was saved.

I pinched myself as my footsteps echoed down the very same corridor leading to the very same ward I knew so well. "I'm here!" I said to myself, "I'll be the best junior doctor they've ever had. I will learn orthopaedic surgery till it's coming out my ears!"

I had a desperate need to say "Thank You" in the best way I could to Professor Robert Roaf, the English surgeon who had operated on me and saved my arm. It was his inspiration and all the experiences during my stay in that hospital that led me to work and study so hard to become a doctor. It was with great emotion and a heart full of thanks that I walked into the same ward, gowned up in the same operating theatre, and took my place at the same operating table where the small miracle was performed for me. Afterwards I wept.

After several more jobs in several more hospitals, I decided a post-graduate degree in the United Kingdom would be my next move. It was a difficult decision to tell my parents that I was going to England. Mum and Dad were

11

very proud that I was going abroad but they wanted me to spend the least amount of time there. I decided I would give it three years, get a Fellowship of the Royal College of Surgeons and then return to India. I also decided to remain single until I had finished my post-graduate degree and had become a fully-fledged surgeon.

I saved enough money to buy an airline ticket to England. I was allowed £3 sterling by the Indian authorities to bring out of the country, so with £3 in my pocket and my suitcase packed, I left for England in June 1966.

The number of people who came to see me off from Palam Airport was overwhelming. I was somewhat embarrassed by all the fuss. After receiving blessings, hugs, garlands and tearful farewells, I left Delhi on a Middle Eastern Airline flight to Bombay. I stayed overnight in Bombay (now Mumbai) in the Sun and Sand Hotel. I had never been inside a hotel before in my life and certainly not a hotel as luxurious as the Sun and Sand.

The doorman, a monumentally tall and magnificent Sikh, in his uniform and turban of royal blue, gold braid on his shoulders and across his expansive chest, saluted me in. A huge chandelier twinkled above the cool and cavernous reception hall. The rich hum of classical sitar music floated on the air and I could see a girl playing it sitting on a floor cushion, her sari draped around her. I caught the fragrance of sweet peas from a large flower arrangement.

My interconnecting flight was from Bombay to Beirut, then a change of airline to Heathrow Airport, London. There were passport check-ups at Heathrow, then a detailed medical check-up during which I had a chest x-ray, and finally I was pronounced medically fit to come into the country.

Upon arrival at Heathrow, I needed the public toilet; misreading the symbols on the door, I went to the ladies. I

12

locked the small cubicle and turned around to see the lavatory seat was raised like a throne. The arrangement was a puzzle to me as I was used to a hole in the ground.

I stood on the seat, balancing with my feet on either side of the pan, and squatted down. On seeing me at the wash hand basins, an indignant woman murmured under her breath whilst some teenage girls giggled behind their hands. One woman, highly offended, tossed her scarf around her neck and set off to find Airport Security!

My cousin Narinder was at the barrier with a "Hey Sat! Over here!" Narinder had been in London for two years working at the Indian High Commission. We took the Tube to his bed-sit in Queensborough Terrace. I was very impressed with the area, which seemed to me at the time very grand with its ornate Georgian architecture. The weather was kind although the sky was grey. A soft drizzle had misted down all night and the temperature was a very pleasant 22C. I was very happy, as I had left 45C in Delhi. The weather was cloudy and overcast, the sort of climate for which England is famous. What a delightful relief from India in June!

After resting for a couple hours, we went out on the town. For me it was an eye-opener. There were no cows, rickshaws or any other transport that I was used to in Delhi. The tall red buses, the elegant black cabs and the beautiful Leyland Mini cars waltzed round the roundabout and travelled up and down the roads in perfect synchrony. I noticed the traffic kept in lanes, in an orderly, well behaved and continuous stream. It stopped at red traffic lights in unison. I noticed it shrieked obediently to a halt if a pedestrian looked as if he *might* just be thinking of crossing the road at a Zebra Crossing.

We strolled together in the soft damp air along Hyde Park Road. We turned in at the gates of the park and took the

13

path to the Serpentine Bar. There we sat at one of the tiny tables overlooking the lake and renewed our friendship over a pint of beer and packets of crisps.

Narinder suggested a walk to The Standard Indian restaurant and then home by way of Bayswater Road. It was Sunday afternoon and there was a street market on the pavement, selling original paintings and antiques. I was fascinated and thought the English very cultured, but I was also surprised to notice beggars in the park approaching passers-by and asking for money. I did not expect to see this in England – particularly London – as I had the impression all the citizens of the country were rich.

Narinder wanted to show me how wonderful his adopted city was. "I'll take you to Speakers' Corner," he said, "You can *really* see free speech in action!" We wandered down to Marble Arch until we came to a number of people clustered around someone standing on a wooden box, shouting, gesticulating and throwing his arms about. He was giving a lecture promoting the Campaign for Nuclear Disarmament. A scuffle broke out amongst some bystanders who did not agree with him. After about fifteen minutes, it all fizzled out and we made our way back to the flat.

On our return, it seemed that many people were going for a walk with a dog on a lead. Dogs were large, medium and small, the miniature ones were sometimes carried like babies in the owner's arms. Dogs were everywhere, soiling the tree trunks and the pavements and I thought: certain things do not change. It does not matter which country you are in.

We sauntered to the shopping area and I could hear horns and see the flashing lights of a police car. I was intrigued to see a group of young ladies in miniskirts: they all looked very attractive. It was the height of summer, so all these ladies were in minimal dresses and their hair was piled high on their heads. Narinder said: "That's what they call a bird's nest hair style."

Near the apartment, we were greeted by one of Narinder's acquaintances. "Good afternoon," he said and lifted his hat to acknowledge us. Narinder said: "Evening, George. Let me introduce my cousin Sat. He is a doctor and has come over to study a bit more. He'll be staying with me for a night or two." The gentleman was a teacher and was interested to hear I had come to do a post-graduation in surgery. He said: "London's recognised as a top-class place for further education, you'll not be disappointed." We talked about education, universities, and the weather; I was having a great time.

When we reached Narinder's apartment, Mrs Jennings, his landlady, invited us in for a drink. This was the first time I had seen a blonde lady at close quarters; she was doubly interesting as she was smoking a cigarette too! She said "I'm what yer call a *proper* Cockney, there's not that many of us left. You could 'ear Bow Bells ringing from me Mum's bedroom winder when I was born. Lived all me life in London, best place in the world!" She talked about all the best places to visit in London. I promised her I would try to see some of this great capital city; but in reality, I knew I was single- minded and focused on achieving the qualification for which I had come.

Three days after arriving in England, I started work as a Senior House Officer in the A&E Department of St Mary's Hospital in Paddington.

There were a number of doctors from overseas in the department and we were left pretty much to our own devices. It concerned me that there were so few doctors and nurses and staff in general. Foreign doctors were invited to come to England for further training, but I quickly realised there was no training plan, we were just an extra pair of hands. As no training programme was evident, we were obliged to pick up informal tutoring from senior colleagues wherever we could, on the ward or in the operating theatre.

A good source of information were the speciality Registrars, if they had a mind to teach us. They also showed us the whereabouts of the plaster room and the blood bank and the correct procedure for filling out forms, and even in which drawer the forms were kept!

My contract was for one hundred and twelve (that is not a misprint: *one hundred and twelve*) hours a week, overtime not included. And, in any case, overtime was not paid extra.

It was assumed at that time that foreign doctors would not fill the more senior positions in the medical profession but return to their own country before becoming eligible to apply for Consultantships. There were three Royal Colleges in the UK: London, Edinburgh and Glasgow. Fellowship or Membership of a Royal College is essential to become a consultant in your chosen speciality. Every consultant must hold a Fellowship or be a Member of one of these three Colleges; my ambition was to pass the exams to become a fellow of the Royal College of Surgeons.

My other mission was a meeting with my hero, the great man who had been there to save me years ago, when my need had been desperate; a man who had, by his skill and experience, set a flame of admiration burning in my heart, a flame that was now a bright and steady fire, an unstoppable force that drove me onward. I needed to meet the source of my inspiration, the reason for my chosen life's work, the man who irrevocably shaped my destiny.

So, on a wet September dawn, I put on my worsted wool grey suit, polished my shoes, Brylcreemed my hair and set off on the early morning train from Euston Station. I arrived at Liverpool Lime Street and walked to The Royal Liverpool Hospital, to meet my hero.

Professor Robert Roaf stood up from behind his desk. It had been seventeen years since he had been in India, but the years had not aged him significantly. He had a few more grey hairs, and his stance was not quite so upright, but his demeanour, the tweed suit, and the twinkle in his eye had not recognised the passage of time at all.

I was a blast from the past. He had pieced together so many smashed limbs, he had drained and cleaned so many infected bones, he had lectured, discussed and debated around the world with leading specialists in all things orthopaedic. He had taught four generations of green, keen young medical students. He had wired and drilled, pinned and plated his way from Liverpool to Lahore and back again. Who *was* this young visitor, who had come so far to say a big *thank you*? In truth, the Professor did not remember me!

Robert Roaf, Professor of Orthopaedic Surgery, cast his mind back to his clinic in the echoing corridors of Irwin Hospital in Delhi, seventeen years before. He *thought* he remembered a man with hopeful eyes, carrying a small boy with an arm so badly infected that maggots crawled in and out of the wound; a boy for whom no more could be done except immediate above-the-elbow amputation and, if he recovered, a false arm, a surgical prosthesis with a hook on the end, provided the family could afford it.

The two of us shook hands and then we melted into a heart-warming, back-slapping hug. Moments like these are rare, they are to be savoured and re-lived again and again. Moments like these, to any doctor, are the perfect result of hard-earned, human efforts to restore health and balance to the human condition. Robert inspected my arm, examined my scars, and tested the movement. As we talked, the professor saw the function he had restored to my fingers, the

17

arm he had drained of pus, and the life he had restored to normality. We talked of my hopes for the future and he saw it was going to be, like his own life, given to the relief of pain and suffering. As the Professor looked at me in the small, cluttered office, the pale northern sunshine streamed in through the window and shone on us both.

India was 6,000 miles away and nearly twenty years ago, but I like to think he saw a reflection of himself in my eyes.

2. Worcester Sauce

AFTER SIX MONTHS serving as a Casualty Officer in Paddington Hospital, I moved to Worcester Royal Infirmary for another six months in Orthopaedic Surgery. In those days, junior doctors covered Casualty (now known as Accident & Emergency) as well as their own specialities. We worked a one-in-two rota (24 hours on, then 24 hours off and so on) including weekends.

Worcester is, of course, a complete contrast to Paddington. "This is *real* English countryside," I thought, "with orchards full of fruit, farming communities and country pubs. There are even great flower beds of Begonias and Lupins in the hospital grounds!" I was keen to learn the flora and fauna, so I bought *The Ladybird Book of British Wildflowers*. I wanted to join in the English way of life, so I noticed that interest in the weather, gardening and horse racing were good topics of conversation, especially as Worcester Royal Infirmary was at the edge of town and very close to Worcester Racecourse.

I felt very comfortable in Worcester; even the doctors' residence was well run and cosy, with dining facilities as if one were in a hotel. We were served typical full English breakfasts, and I was curious to try leek and potato soup, boiled brussels sprouts, pork pies and sausages. The varieties of berries – raspberries, strawberries, blueberries, and redcurrants – were fascinating. The maids were wonderful; and, as they knew we worked upwards of a hundred hours a week, they often said: "Give *me* that laundry, love, I'll run it through the machine for you!" or "Oh doctor, I took those trousers hung over the chair to the dry cleaners, you owe me ten shillings, love."

19

Penelope, a young girl of sixteen, was admitted to my ward having taken a tumble from her horse whilst show jumping. She had sustained a compound fracture of her femur (thigh bone). In the operating theatre, she had the bone pieced together with a metal plate and screws.

Penelope had to remain on the ward in bed for six weeks until the bone had healed over. She was always cheerful, but I noticed that she reserved her brightest smiles for me. She began writing poems which she would press into my hand as I stood beside her bed on ward rounds; the poems often began with: "To Doctor Mehta, Who Makes it Better.'

On her eventual discharge, her parents invited me to their farmhouse for tea; they even came to collect me. The farmhouse and outbuildings stood at the end of a long driveway that swept up to the farmhouse door. Built of stone the colour of warm ochre, the buildings glowed in the afternoon sun. Horses cast long shadows onto the grass beneath, as they silently grazed in the fields surrounding the house.

We took tea on the veranda overlooking the fields, that stretched as far as the eye could see. Tea was an elegant affair with dainty sandwiches, well-risen scones and slices of coffee cake arranged on a three-tier plate which rose high from the centre of the table. A large tea pot and bone china cups rattled on the trolley nearby and Penelope and her parents were the perfect hosts.

Just as I was leaving, I was taken by surprise as they presented me with a tiny white Pekinese puppy as a gift. "He's very cute but I can't accept him," I stammered as they placed him in my arms, "I really don't have the time to look after him, and there's a ban on pets at the hospital residence."

But they ignored my protestations, saying "Now Doctor, what are you going to call him?" They must have thought I was just being polite. "I'll call him Tiger, as he looks so fierce!" I chuckled. So, very reluctantly I brought the puppy to the doctors' residence and asked the maids to help me look after him. In fact, the maids took to the little ball of white fur so much that they adopted him.

I carried on with my duties without worrying, although I knew Tiger's presence in the doctors' residence was against the rules. Peggy, our most "motherly" of maids, eventually took Tiger to live with her. Peggy was a widow, so I like to think Tiger's company was my way of saying "thank you" for all the care she lavished on the junior doctors living so far from home.

The Worcester Racecourse is so close to the Infirmary that by standing in the hospital garden on race days, not only could we hear the horses' hooves as they thundered round the course, but the commentary on the public address system rang out loud and clear. Jockeys regularly attended our Casualty Department with dislocated shoulders, cracked collar bones or concussion. I became accurate and quick at reading x-rays and diagnosing fractures.

The racecourse had a great social life and a thriving pub. Just before closing time, we could occasionally go for a swift lemonade and a packet of crisps, as the bar was within the area that we were obliged to stay when on duty. With no mobile phones in those days, the signalling device we carried, known as a "bleep," operated within a range of 450 metres. The racecourse bar was just within that 450-metre range.

In the department, my opposite number was Clive, a local man whose family owned a farm, growing hops and apples. "Are you doing anything this afternoon, Sat?" he'd say, "Let's hop in the car and go and see Mum and Dad." And with that, we would get in Clive's Mini and were off along the narrow winding country lanes through the lush green Vale of Evesham. Clive's home was a large and picturesque stone farmhouse set in extensive apple orchards and hop-growing fields.

"Great to see you Clive; come in, come in, Sat! It's a pleasure to meet you. Clive told us you work together and get on really well. Come in lads, come in, sit down!" Clive's parents were in their mid-fifties, tall, articulate, and well-spoken. His father had left his wellingtons by the door and was in his stockinged feet, his elegant mother wore a blue tweed dress and jacket and stout leather shoes.

The sunshine streaming in through the window made a lattice pattern on the stone flagged floor. A copper kettle gleamed in the sunlight as it boiled gently on the range cooker. A long low oak table was set with mis-matched china cups and saucers. Huge willow patterned platters filled the dresser set against the wall. Framed sepia photographs of hop-pickers, shire horses and apple orchards were artfully placed on the walls, while from beams above hung bunches of herbs.

"Now lads, tell us what you've been up to," enquired Clive's father as he gestured to us to sit at the table. His mum chuckled as she poured the tea. "Seen any famous jockeys lately? After tea, Clive will show you the farm and you'll be able to taste *real* beer."

I had never seen the way hops are trained to grow in row upon row on 10-foot-high trellises. Casual workers, mostly young people, climbed up to shake the hops down onto mats covering the ground below. The hops were then taken to the barns for adding to the barley mash, yeast, and water. The first beer I ever tasted was brewed on Clive's farm. I found it full bodied, bitter and very enjoyable. I still think beer made with hops is the best beer and bitter is my favourite drink.

When I recall my memories of Worcester, I think of a hospital, clean, well run and a pleasant place in which to serve. I remember the walk along the banks of the River Severn towards Worcester Cathedral. The water shimmered as it flowed silently by, broken only by the cackle of ducks laughing at each other's jokes. Bees and thousands of insects soaked up the juices of grasses and green meadows on hot summer days; by night, the moonlit shadow of the Cathedral reflected in the water and the occasional plop of a water vole or the screech of an owl was the only sound to interrupt my thoughts.

Worcester Cathedral had a close connection with the hospital and its staff. We were often invited for special services and I usually went along. This was my first Christmas, and the Cathedral service was wonderful, the choir sang with great spirit and harmony, the music was inspired, the candles spread a warm glow and the congregation were in festive mood.

But Worcester was not all festivity for me. I was on duty for the Surgical Department every day but had alternate weekends off. I also covered the Accident & Emergency Department at night. There was no supervision in A&E, and I learned to cope on my own very quickly. Senior help would have been a relief, although I would have been better not calling on anyone in *this* case.

One Sunday evening, a woman was found staggering on Malvern Hills. She was confused and wandered into the path of a member of the public and they called an ambulance. When she came in, she lay on the trolley, pale and breathless. She opened her drowsy eyes and told me she had swallowed one hundred and fifty aspirin tablets. The usual dose is no more than 600mg (2 tablets) in six hours, so this was a clear case of aspirin poisoning. I put

23

up an intravenous drip, did stomach washout and, as normal procedure, began arranging her admittance to Ronkswood Hospital on the other side of town. The right medical ward facilities existed at Ronkswood, but I needed to let the Senior Medical Registrar know I was sending her over for overnight observation. My call to the Senior Medical Registrar was logged by the switchboards at both the Infirmary and Ronkswood.

"Hello, Dr Mehta from the Infirmary here, could you put me through to the Senior Medical Registrar on call please? It's urgent."

I was connected through. "Hello. Medical Registrar. What can I do for you?"

I said: "I've got a lady, taken 150 aspirin tablets, 300mg each. I've put up a drip and she's had a stomach washout. I'm sending her over to you to for overnight observation."

"No, mate," he said, "We don't need to admit her, she can go home."

I was taken aback "But she's taken 150 tablets! She's in acidosis! She was found near collapse on Malvern Hills. It's lucky someone found her. She can't go home!"

But he said: "Now look here, sport, we don't need to admit her, that's final!"

I protested that to admit is a normal procedure in all overdose cases, but he put the phone down. I kept the patient for two hours in Casualty; but in the end, I had no option but to discharge her back home in an ambulance. Six hours later, she was brought back to the A&E in a coma; this time she was admitted to Ronkswood Intensive Care Unit, but she died that night. I was very upset that the patient, who should have been admitted and treated many hours before, had now died. But what unfolded next was unbelievable.

It was a sudden death, and so the case was referred to the Coroner. I was asked to give a statement prior to my appearance in court. To my surprise, the Senior Medical Registrar, when he was interviewed by the Hospital Secretary, refused to admit that he had received any call from me. But unbeknown to the Senior Medical Registrar, the Hospital Secretary had contacted both hospital switchboards, and they confirmed that they had logged a call from me to him at the time in question.

Three weeks later, the Coroner's Inquest began. The court assembled: the ambulance staff, the hospital secretaries and the patient's relatives were in court. As the Senior Medical Registrar was not summoned to be in Court, I was amazed to see him there, listening to all I had to say.

The Coroner saw the log of telephone calls put through by both switchboards that night. He found that, on the evidence, I had indeed made that phone call and been refused admission for my patient by the Senior Medical Registrar.

But I felt angry and let down. I went to see my Consultant to tell him about my ordeal. He was incensed and said: "We need to see the Hospital Secretary, Sat. I'll arrange it." Then he added: "Rest assured, action will be taken."

The hospital board sacked the Senior Medical Registrar. The sad details of my patient's death were reported in the local newspaper.

3: Cambridge and Plymouth

AFTER WORCESTER, I was a junior doctor in Cambridge and Plymouth for six months each.

The term *junior doctor* refers to fully qualified doctors who have not become consultants. There are four steps before consultantship, and it took over ten years to progress through the ranks to reach it. Many leave the hospital service along the way. The experience and knowledge gained made the acceptance of total responsibility for everything that took place in your department, easier to shoulder. Now doctors progress much more quickly and specialise much sooner.

Hospital specialities are divided into whichever part of the body or mind is sick; they are further divided into the best way to treat the sickness – with drugs, referring to the medical departments; or with surgery, directed to the surgical departments. A consultant is a specialist in their chosen field. A little bit of history here: Physicians, treating diseases with drugs, retain the prefix Doctor before their name, as years ago they were *the* Doctors. Consultant Surgeons revert to Mister before their name, because before the Royal Colleges were founded, when the Doctor could do no more, the patient might be referred to the Surgeon, who was often the local Barber, as they would have sharp knives and razors!

In Cambridge I was a junior doctor attached to a medical team specialising in heart disease. It was here I learnt to read cardiographs and X-rays of the heart. The department was very busy, so I never had time enough to see Cambridge town.

At Plymouth's Davenport hospital I was again in the medical departments but this time specialising in diseases of the digestive system. The consultant of the department also had beds in the Royal Naval Hospital, and it was here that we treated seafarers who had circumnavigated the globe singlehandedly, but whose digestive systems had suffered as a result of living for months on dried and tinned food.

In the doctors' residence on a fine afternoon, we could assemble a few off-duty colleagues with a "Hey, d'you fancy a trip on the ferry to Saltash Beach?" The fare on the ferry was 6d (old pence) and the beach was a welcome change from the hospital.

However, when my eighteen months experience in the area was finishing, my thoughts turned to the reason I had come so far from home: my quest for admission to the Royal College of Surgeons. I returned to London and stayed in the accommodation apartments at the Royal College to study the course for my Primary Fellowship exam.

The Residency was very luxurious, the dining room was splendidly oak panelled, the tables were laid with white damask tablecloths and serviettes, the glass ware sparkled, and cutlery gleamed. The meals were delicious traditional English fare: we'd have soup, a main course of meat or fish and vegetables, a dessert of stewed fruits or sponge, then cheese and biscuits.

Throughout the meal, red or white wine was served; and with the cheese, the highlight for me was the port, with which we stood, raised our glass in the air as President of the Royal College Professor Lett proposed the toast: "To Her Majesty the Queen!" and we responded: "The Queen!"

There was no television or radio, as it was expected we would be studying hard to pass the exam. I felt privileged to be learning at the College.

I remember Professor Adams from New Zealand, a jolly person who gave the most brilliant after-dinner speeches. "I'll tell you a true story," he began one day, "the

27

story illustrates the power of Mother Love over mere anatomy."

He looked round the room to focus on the ladies. "It happened on a street in Miami, that a toddler ran into the road and was hit by a car. The child lay motionless underneath one of the front wheels of the car. His mother ran into the road and, with no more ado, *lifted* the front of the car off the toddler, whereupon a bystander rescued the child. A check-up at the hospital revealed a bit of bruising, nothing more."

We all sighed with relief. "However," he went on, "The case went to court, the driver of the car saying he never hit the toddler and the mother could not have possibly lifted over a ton of metal off the road. I was asked by the court for an expert opinion, and we ran extensive tests." He grinned. "The tests proved that this 60-kilogram woman, under such extreme circumstances could and *did indeed* lift the front end of the car clear off the road long enough for a bystander to pull the child to safety, on the road that day!"

I also spent hours in the Royal College's Hunterian Museum. The exhibits were gathered initially by John Hunter, an eminent 17th Century surgeon, known for his pioneering work in the ligation of bleeding arteries. In the glass cases I could see how diseases, diagnosis and treatments had evolved over the last three centuries to the present day.

But six weeks is the maximum amount of time the Royal College will allow one to stay, and I had reached that point – so I moved into the YMCA in Tottenham Court Road.

One of the residents in the YMCA was a ballet dancer from South America, training in the Royal Academy. He was small and lithe, and in his shiny black tights and fitted top, he looked like a bendy stick of liquorice. He often entertained us with a dance in the hall, showing us the movements and dress he would wear during his performance. He would suddenly twirl into the dining room and leap with such lightness onto a table. He encouraged all of us to try the same; but, of course, we knew that remaining firmly grounded was our best option. He modelled for us his colourful costumes for his parts in *Harlequin*, *The Firebird* and *Don Quixote*.

Another resident led me to believe he was a professional beggar but, when going out to beg, he was extremely well dressed. I later found out he was a male escort. This was a calling new to me, as I never knew there was such an occupation. He would turn up in the early hours of the morning, aggressive and shouting very abusive language; but he did not want to tell anyone what had happened. We could hear him fumble with his keys in the lock, and stagger into the hallway. "Get out of my fucking way!" he shouted to anyone who opened their door to see what the commotion was. Quite often he would be wearing only one shoe, his trouser zip undone, or his shirt, so clean and smart when he went out, now torn and flapping open. If we showed concern or tried to approach him, he bellowed: "Piss off! Don't come near me!" As he made his unsteady way to his room, we knew we would not see or hear from him again until the next time he went out.

Another student from Eastern Europe was doing a post-graduate course in English Literature and Grammar. He was always talking about Oxford English, Cockney Rhyming Slang and the dialects of Liverpool and Newcastle, which he called Geordie Land. "Aye man, you look a pure belta t'day," he'd say, jerking his head towards the empty chair beside him at the kitchen table, "sit doon an' 'ave a bait wi' me, like!"

Or on the following day his Cockney Rhyming Slang would be "Ah, Sat, pass me that satin and silk (milk) will ya? A 'ad a tumble daan the sink (drink) an got scotch mist (pissed) last night. I'm still feelin' tom and dick (sick)." I don't know how anyone understood him, but he certainly enjoyed straying from Oxford English.

There was also a Scottish pop singer who accompanied himself on his guitar. He wore tight jeans and had blond spiky hair. He sang great songs as he accompanied himself. I saw him a few times busking on the Tottenham Court Road underground. He spoke with a gruff Scottish accent.

You see why I enjoyed staying in the YMCA and meeting young people from all over the world and from all walks of life.

4. Robin Hood Country

IN 1968 I TOOK the post of Casualty Officer in Nottingham General Hospital, a red brick building occupying an elevated site overlooking the city.

On the south side of the hospital is Nottingham Castle with surrounding parklands, and to the north, the old town of Nottingham slopes gently down the hill. A system of underground passages had been hewn in the solid rock, from the medieval Jewish quarter of the town to the castle. The tunnels ran under the hospital and, as luck would have it, a tunnel ran from under the doctors' residence and emerged in two public houses – Ye Olde Salutation and Ye Olde Trip to Jerusalem.

In 1781 the hospital was founded as a charity hospital serving the poor, and in 1948 was assimilated into the NHS. The original building, iron gates and courtyard were still in use, but many extensions had been added over the years. The Casualty Department was opposite the iron gates and opened onto the old courtyard where the ambulances, blue lights flashing, piled in. The Department did not have a dedicated Consultant, but an Orthopaedic Surgeon reputedly ran the place and indeed did turn up occasionally, to see if everything was running smoothly in his absence.

My contract was for five and a half days per week, and night call on alternate nights, making over 100 hours per week. Nottingham Casualty was the second busiest casualty in England. All manner of emergencies – from disastrous coal mining accidents and major motorway smash-ups to kitchen scalds and children's knocks and scrapes – came my way. In the winter months, fractured hip cases filled our female orthopaedic ward beds, as the elderly slipped on icy

31

paths going to the outside lavatory. England still had terrace houses with outside lavatories then. Drunks and drug addicts livened up the weekends.

Most Consultants in those days left emergency night work to be dealt with by their Junior Doctors and were only called from their beds in case of national disaster. We were in at the deep end and we became efficient and well trained. To our patients, we must have looked like sixth formers in white coats, but they had no alternative but to trust us.

It was not unusual for me to attend coal pit disasters and to descend in the cage and crawl down the claustrophobic tunnels to reach the injured. Broken legs and hips, concussion and crushed chests were the usual injuries. I could hear the cries and moans long before I got to the scene. The air would be thick with choking dust and the injured coughed and spluttered out to me exactly where it hurt. The unconscious lay silent under their coating of coal dust. We inserted intravenous drip lines and stretchered them back to the surface. We splinted those with limbs askew and administered morphine to tide them over the journey to hospital. I squeezed back along the mine shaft, up in the cage to the top and took the last ambulance back to the hospital.

Motorbike accidents were the commonest cause of sudden death or injury to young men in those days. I could predict that, over any given weekend, I would send two or three young motorcyclists to the male orthopaedic wards to join the rest of the Royal Enfield, Harley Davidson, Norton, and Triumph enthusiasts.

In the two years I served in Nottingham, I got to know the town well. In the hospital corridor I could be greeted by a fellow junior doctor: "Hey, you off on Wednesday? What say you we see India play West Indies at Trent Bridge?" Or a group of pretty young nurses would say:

"Want to come ice-skating tomorrow afternoon? There's a few of us going, Dr Williams and Dr O'Connor are coming too." The Doctors' Mess was a hive of activity and sport and a melting pot of many nationalities. Alison, our waitress, was more like a mum to us. She made sure we had a clean room, ironed clothes, and a hot meal.

One of the highlights of the year in Nottingham was The Christmas Review Show. It was performed by junior doctors and nurses and ran for three nights. "Hey, Sat!" said Jim, the Rugby-playing hulk of a Medical Registrar, "fancy being my partner in the Review?" Absentmindedly, I assented. "OK," he said, "we've got a rehearsal at eight tonight. See you there."

At one end of the common room in the Doctors' Mess, the rehearsal was in full swing by the time I arrived. Janet, the lovely petite wife of one of the doctors, was demonstrating some delicate ballet steps to the twinkling tune of *The Dance of the Sugar Plum Fairy* from *The Nutcracker*. "Great!" she said when she saw me, "We're all here."

She lined us up in two rows, four big muscular doctors at the back, and in front of them four of us more delicately built men. She tapped a wand and all four of us on the front row were lifted into the air. We twirled and turned and tiptoed our way through to the end of the piece. "Wonderful!" our ballet mistress said with a wan smile, "Needs a bit of work, but we'll have you looking amazing soon.

She then dropped a further bombshell. "I'm getting tights and tu-tus for you all, but I need *you* to beg, borrow or steal a bra and a wig for the next rehearsal on Thursday!" A notice went up in the nurses' home requesting female underwear. We then stuffed the bras with plenty of cotton wool and pulled the tights over our hairy legs. I, being of small stature, had to wear the frilly pink tutu and be tossed through the air by my colleagues.

Jim, my dancing partner, the future Professor of Medicine, was a rugby prop forward and no bra donated by the nurses was big enough to fit him. We could see that the Nurses' Home Sister was well endowed, so we asked to borrow something from her. She gave us a garment that resembled twin hammocks: it would have held up the Forth Bridge, and it fitted Jim admirably. But, unlike the bras donated by the nurses, it had no lace.

We "ballerinas" on the front row were instructed to "tuck in your bottoms and practise your twirls." Whilst the back row had to "lift higher, pass your ballerina up and over your head!"

"Remember," Janet said, flashing her beautiful smile: "you're Christmas Tree Fairies come to life!" Under her long-suffering tutelage we did indeed make some semblance of a ballet troupe, although Tchaikovsky would have wept. We had the distinction of being the most ungainly ballet troupe you would never wish to see – but we brought the house down and were the stars of the show!

In the weeks before Christmas, it became difficult to get into Matron's office past the deliveries from Thresher's off-licence that piled up along her office walls. Staff on duty had to remain *totally sober*, of course. But on Christmas Day off-duty staff turned up to the wards early in the morning to have a drink. It was a busy hospital and, although we tried to discharge as many patients as we could for Christmas, some were too ill for us to do so.

Matron was busy on Christmas Day keeping the balance between the hospital's smooth running in caring for our sick patients and the staff having an enjoyable Christmas. Indeed, the nurses assured me that once you had

had a Christmas in Nottingham General Hospital, you would rather be there than anywhere else!

On Christmas morning, Matron was in the Nurses' Dining Room during their early breakfast, personally giving a small gift to each nurse as they filed past. After that, she invited the medical staff to her office for a drink of sherry. Following tradition, at lunchtime we went back to Matron's office and hoisted her up on our shoulders and carried her to the Nurses' Dining Room. She wore wonderful big pink bloomers. We set her down on the plate-warmer, where she led us in Christmas carols, always ending up with *Silent Night*. Then, as suddenly as it started, it was finished. Matron clapped her hands to bring order to the proceedings, the doctors and nurses sang: "For She's a Jolly Good Fellow!" She dismounted the plate-warmer and, with one final blessing for us all, she was gone.

During the afternoon, those who were off duty dressed in fancy costume and went into the city centre to see the Christmas tree. An off-duty anaesthetist complained he had no fancy clothes to wear so the operating theatre divested him of his clothes and fastened a large terry towel round him as a nappy. A big rubber dummy was put in his mouth and he was wheeled in his pram (a trolley) through the hospital gates and out onto the street, down to the city centre square, to see the Christmas tree.

The tree looked beautiful, so he jumped off the trolley and set about climbing it to get the star at the top. By this time, a crowd had gathered beneath. Unfortunately, halfway up, his nappy began to slip but he had to keep clinging on; and, as it slipped further and further, so the crowd grew. Just as the nappy fell to the ground and he dangled up there in his birthday suit, the police arrived. When he finally came down, we had a police escort back to the hospital. As far as I know, no charges were pressed, and no action was taken.

One of the common emergencies in A&E departments is drunkenness and chronic alcoholism. We had people who regularly turned up blind drunk and paralytic, picked up off the street by the Ambulance Service and brought in on a trolley. We put them on mattresses on the floor, so they did not fall off the trolley if restless or violent. We kept them overnight for observation, so they did not to choke on their vomit.

We also dealt with self-inflicted and sexually motivated injuries. Some of the objects I have removed include a rabbit pelt, bacon rinds, lager and champagne glasses, crayons, children's toys, and electric cables. On one occasion I sent a patient to the operating theatre for removal of a wooden chair leg.

On another occasion, a performer from Nottingham Playhouse came in with abdominal pain. He was dressed in a full-length sequined green gown, high heels, and a long-haired wig. I sensed trouble, so coerced two nurses to come into the cubicle with me. When I examined him, I could find nothing wrong. He just wanted a touch on his body from someone, which is not the purpose of the emergency department. I prescribed a bottle of antacid, reassured him there was nothing seriously wrong and discharged him.

Two ambulance men came into A&E one night and asked that I go out to examine two patients in the ambulance, as they could not be moved. The men would not explain further. In the ambulance I found a young couple lying together on one stretcher. It emerged that, whilst in an amorous and intimate embrace, they had fallen off the sofa and it was feared the young man had sustained such a serious injury as to make separation impossible.

I packed the area with ice and went to see them again after fifteen minutes. We were able to separate them, and we brought them in from the ambulance. I diagnosed a fractured penis and re-packed the area with ice. Eventually we could splint the fracture and they could go home with analgesic tablets.

Nottingham General Hospital was not geared up to dealing with the delivery of babies. In those days it was not uncommon that young girls who had accidently become pregnant were too afraid to tell their parents or their GP. When "abdominal pains" began, they would be brought to the Hospital, arriving often in the later stages of labour. We sometimes delivered babies either in A&E or even in the ambulance. We would then transfer the mother and child and the shocked grandparents to the Women's Hospital on the other side of town.

One day a patient came who was clearly in labour. I determined that we had time to transfer her to the Women's Hospital, but I wanted a qualified midwife from amongst our staff to travel with her. The Nursing Sister who could go, I knew well: she was a highly qualified midwife and was charming, but shy and easily embarrassed. When she bustled in, I instructed her earnestly: "Now, Sister, I think you'll have time to get there. But if she starts pushing in the ambulance, I'll give you this big roll of Elastoplast to dam things back, OK?" She nodded gravely; but when she arrived at the Women's Hospital, she relayed my instructions to the Midwives there. They immediately burst into peals of laughter. She returned to A&E, stormed up to my desk and threw the roll of Elastoplast at me. I was very nearly a casualty myself that night.

A large Polish man was carried in one day by two of his work colleagues. They were working on a building site when he had caught his arm in machinery. The two friends had made a sling but said it was a wonder he had an arm still attached to him. His agonising screams boomed loud in the department and down the nearby corridors. Casualty Sister was frantic and wanted me to see him urgently.

The patient had a dislocated shoulder, his arm hung uselessly out of its socket. It needed to be reduced quickly, otherwise the muscle would go into spasm and reduction of the dislocation would be much harder, requiring a muscle relaxant.

I felt confident enough to reduce the dislocation and knew that most Casualty staff would never again have a chance to see the manoeuvres I was about to do. I summoned all available staff to the Minor Operating Theatres, and I got our very muscular patient to sit on the edge of the operating table. A half dozen staff hurried to the theatre and waited expectantly to see how this miracle was performed. I positioned myself behind the patient and pulled his arm backwards and then straight out at right angles. We all heard a loud click; the shoulder went back into its socket and suddenly he was completely pain-free.

The patient beamed in delight. First, he hugged me, then covered me in kisses "Oooh! Doctor, YOU good, GOOD man!" He lifted me into the air and hugged me to his chest, so my legs dangled off the ground. The nurses grinned, enjoying my plight, folded their arms and did nothing to help me!

5. Doctor in Danger

I TOOK OVER the Casualty department one Saturday night and all was relatively quiet. Night staff are used to working in bursts of extremes, extremely tranquil or relentlessly hectic. After 8pm, hospitals put fewer staff on duty because routine cases are seen during the day and only emergencies are brought in at night.

Up until midnight, we had a woman having her scalded hand dressed, a merrily drunk young man having his broken ankle plastered and a drowsy young girl being transferred to a medical ward following her tranquilliser overdose.

But at about half past midnight, the entrance doors flew open, and two ambulance men appeared dragging a violent drunk to a mattress on the floor. We always put drunks on the floor as we found they tended to scramble off trolleys and land up on the floor anyway. The patient was large, bulky, sweating and abusively loud. The ambulance men, muscular and strong themselves, had clearly had a struggle with him in the ambulance.

The patient was accompanied by a dishevelled looking man and a girl, whom we conducted to waiting room chairs. "Fuck off!" the patient roared, "You get off me!" He was all elbows and knees, as he lashed out at anyone who came within striking distance. A chair went flying across the room and staff nurse dodged a punch at her face. Our hospital porter, staff nurse, student nurse, and I joined the two ambulance drivers in getting the patient onto a mattress.

"Fuck you!!" he spat, as he kicked one foot towards the ceiling, and the other foot he directed at my ribs. I heard a loud crack and immediately had a searing pain in my chest.

I decided we had to control him as fast as possible, so I sent staff nurse to draw up a syringe of Paraldehyde. The drug is a powerful sedative but is so corrosive to muscle that it must be given deep into the buttock muscle and in a glass syringe, as it melts a plastic one. Even then, the drug took an hour to work.

"Here, Doctor Mehta, take these," said Staff nurse, as she handed me two DF118 (strong painkillers) and a cup of tea. At 2am we sent the patient, sleeping soundly, to the ward. I carried on until the X-Ray department opened in the morning. Three cracked ribs showed on the X-ray films and there was extensive bruising to my chest and arm. The cracked ribs made expanding my rib cage to draw each breath very painful, so I took DF118 for three weeks. The tenderness lasted for a year and the legacy is a dull ache that returns during very cold or damp weather.

Medical staff are often vulnerable to physical attack. At one time, I was working in a Birmingham Hospital; and, to earn a bit of extra money, I signed up with the Locum Deputising Service. The majority of general practitioners now use these Deputising Services to attend their out-of-hours emergency calls.

My sessions started at 8pm and finished at 2am. My wife Kate, armed with a map and a flask of tea, often came with me in the car; but, since we had a baby by then, that was no longer possible. I had been very busy all night, and this last call was at about half past midnight.

The call was to see a lady in a run-down area of Birmingham, a maze of back-to-back terrace houses with metal bars at the windows and doors. Scattered along the pavements were dustbins, litter and empty bottles and street lights lit the road only dimly. I was looking for house numbers, usually scrawled in dripped, chipped and faded paint on the doors, walls, or anything else to hand. The only life on the street was a barking dog and a drunk, swaying dangerously into the road.

The patient had rung her GP's emergency number to ask for a home visit because she was suffering from varicose veins. The veins, she said, were causing itching to the skin on her ankles and her boyfriend was very concerned and wanted her to be admitted to the hospital.

I found the house and knocked; eventually the door was flung open by a large unshaven man wearing a string vest. The hallway was dark, and I noticed the door to the yard at the back was nailed shut. In the sitting room the patient lay on a settee; cigarette smoke rose from her ashtray on the floor. As I bent over to examine her legs, a large hairy arm, belonging to the patient's boyfriend, jabbed my shoulder as he roared "She's needin' the 'ospital! I'm sick of 'er moanin'."

I said: "Varicose veins is not an emergency." I continued: "Excuse me, while I talk to the *patient*." I examined her abdomen and talked to her in detail concerning her problems. I suggested I get in touch with her GP so that she could be seen in the hospital by a Vascular Surgeon and have a Doppler Scan on her varicose veins.

Both the patient and her boyfriend were covered in tattoos. The boyfriend had a scorpion on his chest and serpents coiled down his arms. He had a revolver on his neck, a dragon on his back and a small hammer on his forehead. The patient had butterflies and flowers on her thighs.

The boyfriend became angry and started shouting: "I don't want 'er in the 'ouse! She fucking needs the 'ospital!" I pulled myself up to my full five-foot-five-inches and said: "The hospital is sleeping at the moment. She needs to be referred by her GP to a Vascular Surgeon and any further action will be taken from there." His eyes blazed as he swayed about the room, belching and scratching his scorpion. He lunged forward and pushed me against the wall, "Ya STILL don't fuckin' understand, do ya! We need to do something NOW! Else YOU won't be leaving 'ere! Ya NOT getting out of 'ere till ya take 'er with ya!"

I was alarmed and frightened by his attitude, but I tried to calm him, saying: "What I'm telling you is the best route to take. The appointment can be made by your GP to see a surgeon and to proceed from there."

He thumped me on my head and shoulders and pushed me into the back of the house against the nailed-up door. My mind was racing, as I could see no way out. He stood between me and the front door. I was there for three quarters of an hour, trying to reason with him while he thumped and slapped me around.

"This will not solve the problem. Even if you ring the hospital for admission, they will not accept you in the middle of the night," I told the patient.

Eventually she screamed: "Buzz! Buzz! It ain't goin' nowhere!" She rose from her settee and said, "I'm going to the doctor first thing. *He'll* get me in." She lit another cigarette and said: "These little scruffs, they don't know *nothin'*." So Buzz grabbed me by the back of my jacket and threw me out on the street.

Trembling and shaken, I found a telephone kiosk and rang Kate. When I arrived home, Kate was waiting with strong sweet tea and a brandy. "That's it!! No more deputising!" she said, "I don't care what you've got booked in tomorrow night, you resign as from now!"

Kate was adamant. I was very upset and could not sleep properly. The following morning, I rang the manager at the deputizing service. I told him what had happened. I explained that the woman should be put on a register so that any doctor visiting her would be accompanied. I told him he

42

should also get in touch with her GP. I gave him my resignation.

The following week, the Deputising Service Manager asked to come over to our house because he wanted to speak to us personally. "I've come to tell you the sequel to that visit," he said, "After you left, he strangled her to death!" Kate and I gasped. He went on: "*She's* dead and *he's* in custody." The manager asked me to re-consider my resignation, so I signed up again – but insisted I do only day-time visits and accompanied by a driver at all times.

But this was not the only violence I encountered in Birmingham. On the evening of 21 November 1974 around 8pm, I was on duty at the General Hospital when a call came through that a major incident had happened in the city centre. Two huge explosions had blown up The Tavern in the Town and The Mulberry Bush public houses. We had to prepare for catastrophic injuries. The police sealed off the whole city centre and no-one was allowed in or out of the area. All telephone calls were forbidden, so Kate heard about the explosion on the local radio and knew I would not be home for some time.

The IRA had planted three bombs, two had exploded and one remained unexploded somewhere in the city centre. The bombers had apparently tried to warn the pubs that an explosion was imminent, but every telephone kiosk they tried in Birmingham had been vandalised, so no warning came.

The victims started to arrive, hurried in on trolleys, blood-soaked and unconscious; they arrived on foot, covered in white plaster dust, speechless and bewildered. They arrived with limbs, eyes and hair missing. We put pity to one side and swung into action. The final toll was 21 dead and 180 seriously injured. Kate watched the TV in horror as police swarmed all over the city centre. Blue lights flashed and sirens blared, and ambulances were engaged in an endless ferrying to the hospital and back again.

It emerged later that a third bomb had been planted outside Barclays Bank but did not go off. The IRA claimed responsibility for the bombings.

Six suspects were arrested, convicted and sentenced to life imprisonment in 1975. In 1991, on appeal, their conviction was declared unsafe and unsatisfactory and they were released. The actual bombers were promised anonymity and received an amnesty as part of the Good Friday Agreement.

6. A Very English Romance

IT WAS THE USUAL busy Saturday night in the Casualty Department of Nottingham General Hospital. In the curtained-off bays lay a young girl having her stomach pumped of the barbiturate tablets she had taken, an elderly lady who had gone down her garden path to the outside toilet, slipped and fractured her femur, so I had ordered an X-ray then admittance to the orthopaedic ward. In the next couple of bays were two car passengers with head injuries from a road traffic accident, who would also have to be admitted for observation, and next to them, a collier from the coal mine with two sawn off fingers in a plastic bag full of ice, and finally a woman in labour, who would be going shortly to the Women's Hospital.

We never needed a clock to know when closing time at the pub was… the intoxicated started rolling in within half an hour, and that time had come. The ambulance men brought them in two or three at a time. As they came in, they were laid on the floor around the walls of the department, on blue plastic covered mattresses. In this way they could not roll off a trolley.

I checked and dealt with any injuries and then either admitted them to a ward or kept them on the mattresses until sober. It was under these circumstances that I caught a glimpse of my future wife.

Rita, a poor unfortunate vagabond well known to us, had been brought in having consumed a great deal of alcohol: it might have been gin or methylated spirit. She had fallen in the River Trent. She was rescued by a passer-by and brought in by the Police. Soaking wet and smelling of alcohol and vomit, she protested loudly as we wrapped a

45

blanket around her and laid her on a mattress. She was covered in mud and blood, so a lovely little nurse I had not seen before set to work with a bowl of hot water, a flannel and towel. I could then see Rita's many lacerations and from where the blood was coming.

Rita protested with colourful language while I stitched her wounds, so two nurses held her fast, until I had completed the job. I then left instructions that she was to have an Anti-Tetanus injection and an injection of Penidural, a short-and-long-acting Penicillin. Penidural is a very effective antibiotic and only needs the one dose; however, it is the consistency of thick treacle and must be given by deep intra-muscular injection, into the buttock.

Shortly afterwards I was attending to another patient when I heard loud screams and shrill curses coming from Rita's corner on the floor. I swirled around to see a fight, furious and thrashing, a wrestling match of arms and legs rolling all over the department floor. A starched white but crumpled apron and cap, then a muddy leg and blanket, now a mud-stained bottom and torn wet skirt. The pretty little nurse had been sent to give Rita her injections, but Rita was having none, of it.

I was enjoying assessing the situation, when what came next nearly sent me heading for the cardiac arrest trolley. A flash of black stockings and the most, lovely silky thighs and suspenders! I nearly fainted with delight. Agitated and hot, I decided to fetch our three large and trusty Casualty Porters. I hurried to get them, and they went to their task with gusto. Rita had her injections, and I had my interest piqued.

After that, I sought the pretty nurse out to help me whenever I could. I learnt her name was Kate and she was nineteen. She told me that normally only student nurses in their third year of training are sent to Casualty. Kate was only in her second year. Nottingham Casualty had a fearsome reputation on many counts. It was the second busiest Casualty in the country (Birmingham being the busiest). And it was reputed to have powerful effects on the nurses, "A stint in Nottingham Casualty," they said, "changes you forever, you either end up drinking, smoking, gambling, or married."

Kate and I had the same values and outlook on life, so the fact that we were from different backgrounds, religious faiths and countries did not overly concern us. Ours was not an intense and starry-eyed affair. I felt grounded and easy in her company and could see that a future together would be very happy.

When our erratic off-duty hours coincided, we spent them together. In the early hours of the morning, we often dropped into the transport café at Trowell Service Station on the M1 motorway – not the most exotic of venues, but open 24 hours. I was preparing to do my Fellowship exams and studying hard. We both knew the whole purpose of my being in the UK was to become a Fellow of the Royal College of Surgeons, but it came as a surprise when one day Kate said: "I've been thinking. We've known each other for more than a year now..." She looked at me intently. "I'm sure about *you*, but if you're not sure about *me*, I'm ending the relationship now!" I was astonished. "A year is enough for anyone," she went on "we either get engaged or I'm off!" She smiled sweetly and waited for my answer.

"Well," I stammered, "There's my exams coming up!"

She smiled again "Yes, I know. Engagement doesn't stop you studying; in fact, it should help." I could see she really had thought it through whilst I had just cruised along, enjoying the relationship as it was. "It's no problem," she said as she rose from the table, "I'll not waste any more of your time. If you don't know now, you never will."

Clearly, there was only one thing for it. Derby Road in Nottingham is well known for its many antique and jewellery shops. Kate had seen a small diamond ring that she liked in Woodward's Jewellers: it had five small diamonds set in rose gold and it came in a heart-shaped box. We bought the ring, and I made a date to take her out to dinner.

Kate had quite often eaten dinner in the hospital when she came off duty, but nevertheless was ready for another with me later in the evening. "Give her up, she's too expensive!" my friend Oliver often advised, "She *always* wants feeding!" I arranged a taxi to take us to The Château Restaurant near the Trent River. I bought a red rose and had the ring in my pocket. Before dessert, I suddenly pushed my chair aside and got down on one knee "Will you marry me?" I asked, as I produced the box from my pocket.

Kate said "Yes!" and beamed with her beautiful eyes. We clinked our wine glasses, and I slipped the ring on her finger.

"Congratulations!" The diners on the next table toasted us with raised wine glasses, and we grinned at all around us. It was a fantastic evening as we walked along the River near Trent Bridge.

After a few weeks, Kate suggested I should meet her parents to ask their blessing and approval. So, on a fine spring morning, we set off by bus to Grantham and then boarded another bus to Donington. We walked two miles to get to the village where she lived. The house was a large white house built in the 18th Century. It was surrounded by a lush green garden and bounded by tall shady trees, a lawn at the front and a further lawn and orchard at the back. I felt this was to be a momentous occasion. We opened the door and stepped into the kitchen: here her parents stood, and I immediately had an uneasy feeling. Tony, Kate's father, was tall, dark, slim and classically handsome and, as Kate formally introduced me, he extended his hand, but a smile did not reach his eyes "How do you do? Have you had a pleasant journey?" he enquired.

Her mother Anne was reticent but polite. She had a lovely Scottish accent and her twinkly blue eyes danced as she said "Ah, you'd both like a cup of tea right now?" We sat in the oak-beamed dining room, "Where do you want Sat-y-aa to sit ?" enquired Kate's father (My full first name is Satya.)

"Next to Kathleen," her mum replied. We drank tea and ate a delicious ham and salad meal. It was a lovely summer evening; so, after tea, Kate and I escaped into the garden and she showed me where she used to play under the lush green boughs of the tallest chestnut trees in Lincolnshire!

There was an old tractor cabin that had made her and her two sisters a splendid playhouse. We peeped into three ancient pan-tiled outhouses and then went for a walk through the adjoining fields, stretching, as fenland fields do, to beyond the horizon. We walked until dusk and then turned for home.

"And now, Sat-y-aa" said Kate's father, "I'll show you to your rhuum." He pronounced room with a *rhu* sound, which sounded very grand. I followed him up the creaking stairs and, as he opened the door to a pleasant room, a tall grandfather clock directly outside on the landing chimed. "Ahh, strikes every quarter hour, hope it won't disturb you."

I put my small bag on the bed and went back downstairs for another hour. They had retired to the sitting room where they were engrossed in the TV programmes until bedtime at 10pm. The following morning Kate and I, after a fantastic typical English breakfast, set off on the two-mile walk to the next village to catch the bus to Grantham, and then another onto Nottingham. Kate's parents were displeased with our relationship. Kate was not surprised at her parents' disapproval, and my own parents had also remained silent on the subject which we interpreted as their dissatisfaction also.

Returning to Nottingham, I invited my friend Oliver for drinks in the Doctors' Mess and we discussed my visit to my future in-laws. "Sat," he said after a great gulp of bitter, "Why are you bothering?" He frowned. "It's more trouble than it's worth, mate. Anyway, if I know women, which I don't, Kate might dump you if her parents make life so unhappy for her. Besides, she's a Roman Catholic, isn't she? And you're Hindu! Bet you didn't drop *that* bombshell!" Oliver was warming to his advice. "Think, man! Your kids will never be accepted. No!" He shook his head sadly. "It'll be troubling all your life. If you want my opinion, mate, it's a non-starter."

On her next nights off, Kate made another brief visit to her parents "Your father and I want you to wait a year," advised her mother, "If he's still around, we'll see then."

"Yes, that we can do. What's a year out of a lifetime?" Kate reassured her parents, so we delayed our plans and promised not to marry for a year.

Sadly, during that year, Kate's parents did not contact her. When she went to see them on her 21st birthday, they gave her a card, but unsigned by anyone. Although I was very upset by the way we were treated, Kate seemed remarkably undeterred and calm.

As I said before, whenever our off-duty coincided, we spent time together. However, I applied for a surgical job in Stoke-on-Trent. It was a move I had to make to get more experience and get ready to do my Fellowship exam. I also thought that, as we were apart, our relationship would be tested, and we would see if it was strong enough to withstand separation. I took driving lessons and bought a little red VW Beetle car so that I was able to visit Nottingham on my weekends off. We had a wonderful time together whenever we met.

I bought Kate a lovely gold bracelet and could not wait to present it to her. I waited near the Nurses' Home and eventually she came down the pathway towards me. "Come," she said, "We'll go to The Bramcote Room. I can make you a cup of tea there." No visitors were allowed inside the Nurses' Home, especially young men, so the Bramcote Room, a small annexe where nurses could entertain their visitors, was where we went. The Bramcote Room had an enormous bay window with a direct view of the hospital back gates. Hospital Staff used the back gates and had a clear view, through the bay window.

My new Consultant at Stoke was an ardent football fan and a Director of Stoke City Football Club. They were in the First Division at that time and we sometimes saw players who turned up unexpectedly for medical treatment.

I knuckled down to my Fellowship studies in earnest. The first part of my exam was in Dublin. I had a few friends who had also entered for the exam, so off we went together. When I rang the college a week or so later for the exam result, I found I had passed! So had my friends!

"I knew you'd do it!" Kate enthused over the phone, "Have you sent an airmail letter to your Mum and Dad? Better still, could you phone their next-door neighbour and ask to talk to them?" Mum & Dad did not have a phone in the house, but the next-door neighbour did. We celebrated with a drink the next time we got together in the little bar in Nottingham Playhouse.

Kate had passed her exam also and was now a qualified State Registered Nurse. She was on night duty and ran Nottingham's five Emergency Operating Theatres. Working eight twelve-hour night shifts gave her six full days off, during which she came to stay in the guest room in Stoke.

She telephoned her parents to say the year's delay was nearly up and we had faithfully kept our part of the agreement.

Her parents said something like: "If you marry *that man*, you need never darken our doorstep again!"

Kate replied: "I'm sorry you feel like that. I know you only want the best for me, but we've kept our part. I've never hidden anything from you and we're still together. So now we'll go ahead."

There was silence from the other end of the phone, then they put it down. When two years had elapsed and their stance had not changed, we got engaged and decided to marry in Nottingham Cathedral.

Most of my hospital friends, even Oliver, were very supportive and said: "We'll be there on your wedding day!" Kate's friends also gave her their full support and blessing and promised to attend our wedding. And there were even a few who wanted to take her down the aisle for the ceremony.

We went to Nottingham Cathedral and arranged a date for the wedding. I also signed up for the pre-wedding course, detailing exactly what marrying a Roman Catholic would entail. "The Mass is the most important part, and your nuptials are only part of it," said the priest. He was very helpful and happy to guide me in the Catholic faith but told me strongly: "When you have children, they must be baptised in the Church and you will bring them up in the one true Catholic Faith. Furthermore, you should provide them with a Catholic education in a Catholic school".

The Albany Hotel near both the Cathedral and Hospital was well known for hosting wedding receptions so we arranged the reception there.

Kate said: "Don't you think it's about time you informed your own parents?" I had been in touch with my parents regularly since coming to the UK and had mentioned Kate as my very close friend. I subsequently sent detailed letters about Kate and enclosed photographs, eventually saying we were engaged and planning to get married. There was a deafening silence. I did not receive a letter for two months. But eventually my father wrote a very congratulatory and welcome letter to Kate and me and gave us their blessing. I was over the moon to know they were pleased with my decision, even though I knew my mother had in mind three Indian lady doctors whom she considered suitable for me to marry.

Kate and her friends qualified as State Registered Nurses in September of 1969. When they began training, they were 18 years old and in law, still minors. Their parents had entrusted them to the hospital's safekeeping. Now they were all 21 years old and legally adult. Eager to be independent, she and five of her friends moved out of the Nurses' Home and rented a house on Nuttal Road.

It was around Christmas when I motored down to the new house to see Kate. She had mentioned to her friends that Stoke Hospital did not have the riotous Christmas that Nottingham enjoyed; so, knowing I was expected any minute to collect her, they kindly said: "Aah, poor Sat, we'll soon fix that." And they ran upstairs to prepare a bath full of warm water topped off with a large amount of foam. They were waiting for me behind the front door. I was pushed, pulled and bodily lifted up the stairs and plunged into the bath. I managed to pull three girls in with me as water and foam covered the floor.

But the girls, always careful not to overdo things, provided me with a towel when I scrambled out and suggested my trousers hang on the kitchen pulley to dry.

Just then the doorbell rang, and Kate's parents stood glowering on the doorstep. They were paying a surprise visit, they said, and they asked was Kathleen in? Luckily, she had remained dry and went down to greet them. Kate and two dry friends entertained them with tea and biscuits, as if nothing at all was happening upstairs. The only give-away was my dripping trousers hanging on the kitchen pulley.

Suddenly they noticed the engagement ring on Kate's finger "What's that?" they exclaimed. So Kate explained we were getting married in Nottingham Cathedral and arrangements were at an advanced stage.

They were very displeased but avoided another confrontation. Kate told me later that, on their return home, her father had said: "Are you thinking what I'm thinking?" And her mum said: "Yes. If the Church is willing to marry them, who are we to disagree?" Two weeks later Kate received a letter from her Father, saying they accepted our marriage and invited us to get married in Spalding church.

7. Wedding Bells

WE VISITED KATE'S PARENTS so I could officially ask their belated permission and blessing to marry. "Sat," said Kate, before we arrived, "Comment on the eight big chestnut trees at the *front* of the house, that should win Dad round, he is very proud of them, they're the tallest Chestnut Trees in Lincolnshire. In fact, our house is called The Chestnuts."

I remembered Kate's advice as Tony and I walked round and round the back lawn. I pointed to the row of poplar trees and, as we passed the open kitchen window, Kate groaned as she heard me say: "They're lovely chestnut trees, Dad."

I asked if he had any advice on marriage to give. He thought for a moment and said with a grin: "Yes. Keep a dog – they're always faithful."

So we were welcomed into the family and arrangements were made for us to get married in the Catholic Church in Spalding with a wedding Reception afterwards at Springfield's Restaurant and Conference Centre. I was invited to visit them again to see the Priest and acquaint myself once again with my part during the ceremony. We had 80 guests at our wedding day. I had no direct family members except my cousin Narinder and Eva, his Dutch wife. Most of the guests on my side were my medical or nursing colleagues. Most of Kate's guests were family members: uncles, aunts, cousins, and her grandma.

Two days before the wedding, I invited my friends to a pub on the main road near Stoke City Hospital and we continued afterwards in the bar in the hospital mess. We had a great time with singing and dancing. I was properly drunk, and my friends had to carry me to my bed. In fact, I was legless. I can't remember much except that I was constantly sick; and in the morning, I couldn't get out of bed. A friend came over to check if I was fit enough to come on the Ward Round. He decided I was dehydrated so he went to the ward, gathered some equipment, and put an intravenous drip into me. He joked: 'We may just have to walk you up the aisle hooked up to this drip!"

I spent a few more hours in bed but recovered enough to drive my VW Beetle to Nottingham and from there my best man Oliver– the same Oliver who had advised me not to get married – drove to Kate's parents' house, the same large two-hundred-year-old farmhouse surrounded by beautiful gardens in the tiny village of Quadring, in the flat farmlands of the Lincolnshire Fens. We spent a while talking with Kate's parents on the back lawn and then, late in the evening, we booked into the Red Lion Hotel and turned in for the night. I prepared my wedding speech late that night, from a book.

We were married on a sunny summer morning in July 1970. Oliver drove me to St Norbert's Catholic Church. I was still suffering the effects of my stag night two nights previously, so I had an upset stomach and a headache.

Kate came down the aisle on the arm of her dad. She came and stood by my side whilst *Ave Maria* played on the church organ. She wore a simple silk gown and long veil. I was mesmerised.

The reception was held in the function room in Springfields Centre in Spalding. I was introduced to Kate's wonderful grandma, whom everyone knew as Mopsy. She was resplendent in her hat with an ostrich feather round the crown, which gently caught the breeze. She held a fluffy Pekinese dog in her arms. Mopsy had a twinkle in her eye as she said, "I'm very pleased to meet you, Satya. I'm happy you are bringing new blood into the family." I introduced myself to the rest of Kate's family, including Kate's Scottish side: her three aunts and two uncles. They were very jolly, and it was lovely to see everybody enjoying the occasion. My father-in-law made a speech, and I thanked all my guests and remembered my parents many miles away. My best man Oliver read telegrams from my parents and relations in India. The reception finished about four o'clock in the afternoon. Kate went to get changed out of her wedding dress and I went to get my car.

I hardly recognised my little red Beetle, decorated as it was in ribbons and streamers. In big daubs of window cleaner on the doors was scrawled *Once a King, always a King, but once a Knight's enough!* My new mother-in-law was scandalised. The boot said *Just Married* and pennies in the wheel hubs whizzed round and round with a loud rattle. It was a car that drew cheers and waves as we chugged up the A1 motorway. The first thing we bought, as Mr and Mrs Mehta, was an ice cream at a motorway service station. In London, we arrived at The Cumberland Hotel in Marble Arch. We met up with Narinder and Eva and enjoyed a meal and a great evening in London together, before they took their flight back to the Netherlands.

It was our first night together as Mr and Mrs. As we settled down into the bed, I noticed a sign on the headboard saying: *Massage Boy* and below it a large red button. I said to Kate: "Why don't we press the button?" She said: "No young lad is coming into our room to give *me* a massage!" It was, of course, simply a massaging mechanism on the bed. Years later, I teased Kate about it, but it would have been more than my life was worth to tease her then.

The next day we enjoyed the sites of London as we drove the car, still decorated, over Chelsea Bridge and London Bridge and parked near Hyde Park.

Unknown to Kate, I had taken out a bank loan and booked a surprise honeymoon in Switzerland. Our hotel in Montreux, on the banks of Lake Geneva, was an ancient stone edifice, transformed into a luxurious hotel. Our room, with eighteen-inch-thick walls, had wooden shutters at the mullioned windows. We took breakfast each morning in our room at a little table under the window, spread with starched damask linen, looking out onto shimmering Lake Geneva. The hotel's lift was a very ornate wrought iron one that carried no more than four passengers. The dining room was the only modern extension to the hotel, comprising a curved glass wall overlooking the lake, and behind, near the entrance, a large door that presumably led to the kitchen.

We took a trip to see nearby Chillon Castle, where in 1532 the monk, Francois Bonivard was imprisoned. Lord Byron famously took up the story when, in 1816, he wrote: "My hair is white, but not with years/ Nor grew it white in a single night/ As men's have grown from sudden fears." It ends: "My very chains and I grew friends./ So much a long communion tends/ To make us what we are: even I/ Regain'd my freedom with a sigh."

Next day we rode the little rack and pinion train, up through the sweetly perfumed meadows dotted with alpine flowers, to above the snowline and onto the Great St Bernard Pass and the Monastery. The dogs, for which the monastery is famous, looked as big as miniature ponies and well enough covered in long thick fur to withstand the winters up there. There were plenty of chubby, round puppies, tumbling, rolling, and yelping amongst the straw of their large compound. We stayed for a few hours, had a beer and some salad, and admired the view of the Alps from a little restaurant high up in the mountains. We chose a table outside, despite the wind, on account of the beautiful view of the valley far below. A sudden gust of wind blew a lettuce leaf off Kate's plate and up into the air. I sprang up and ran after it, but the lettuce spiralled up, up and away, over the mountain tops and away into Italy.

Lake Geneva looked tempting, so we hired a boat for a couple of hours. We started well and got to the other side of the lake. Trouble was, I could not turn the boat around to head back. Our two-hour slot came and went. Kate could see how to reverse the engine and turn the boat around, but to spare my feelings she avoided giving a hand to my mechanical skills. Towards evening, we were racking up the hire fee and we were getting hungry. So in the end Kate did something with the outboard motor, turned the boat around and brought us back.

I wanted to show my new wife a good time and took her to a nightclub. I sat with my back to the stage and my beautiful wife sat opposite, facing the stage. I had not researched the venue well enough. When the curtains flew back and the show started, Kate was not amused that I had taken her to a cabaret show on the same lines as the Folies Bergère in Paris. It was interesting for me though.

Before the wedding, I had discussed the honeymoon with Kate's mum and had mentioned a few European countries under consideration but had not finalised the holiday at the time. It was nice to see an article in the *Spalding Guardian* that said we had honeymooned in Switzerland, France and Italy, a grand tour of Europe according to my new in-laws!

We arrived back to live in a ground floor flat in Stoke. Kate took a job as staff nurse in the operating theatre. To celebrate our new apartment, I posted on the hospital noticeboard that we were holding a housewarming party. "How many's coming?" asked Kate,

"Oh, a few," I shrugged. In the event, *one hundred and fifty people* turned up bearing drinks, food, plates, and bed rolls. I invited all our neighbours in the street too.

Married life was wonderful, and we still had lovely lunches as Kate wanted to carry on where the hotel left off. We even had a half bottle of wine with our evening meal! We were enjoying life, looking after each other and attending parties and other invitations extended by our new friends. I now felt part of society and of the church and proud to talk about England as my home. After our marriage, my loneliness had gone. I had got myself a partner. That added everything to my life, and I started supporting England at international games and sports!

Then Kate announced, to our great happiness, that she was pregnant. She gave up work and spent her time in the apartment. She began to be lonely. We decided she should have a pet for company. So it was that Charlotte, our beloved Cairn terrier puppy, came to live with us. Charlotte was very playful, but when tired would climb into my coat, so her head rested on my chest and thus she accompanied us everywhere. I often took her to be doctors' bar in the common room to meet my friends. On one occasion a saucer of beer was put down for her and very soon she began to stagger on her short tubby legs; she really could not walk in a straight line. When we got home, I was in trouble with Kate for getting Charlotte drunk. We gently put her in her basket where she stayed for the next 24 hours, no doubt with a thumping headache.

I was finishing my job in Neurosurgery and I wanted to get back into General Surgery. As luck would have it, we were invited to a hospital dinner party and so it was that Kate sat next to an eminent ear nose and throat (ENT) surgeon. During their conversation, Kate raised the point that I was likely to get stuck in the job's "bottleneck". They discussed

60

the possibility of my switching to ENT, there being more prospect of promotion in that branch. "Why doesn't he come and work for me?" he suggested. In discussion with Kate later that night, we decided that I should take up his offer and switch. I would have to take demotion from Registrar to Senior House Officer, but, if all went well, this would not be for long.

This was a complete change for me, and I have been grateful to Kate ever since for helping me switch my speciality. My wide experience in medicine, surgery and trauma has proved invaluable in giving me insight. If my patients' symptoms don't add up, I can investigate areas other than my own speciality.

I took up my new ENT post in Birmingham in 1971. We were given hospital accommodation: the ground floor flat in a large draughty house in Handsworth. Once a grand town house, it had seen better days. The accommodation was not satisfactory but, as we were expecting a baby, we decided not to move.

My hospital was in Birmingham city centre. I was on call alternate nights and alternate weekends. So, three days and nights during the week and every other weekend, from Friday morning through to Monday night, I was obliged not to leave the hospital premises. In those days there were no mobile phones and Kate did not drive. It was not satisfactory, but we had to put up with it.

8. Lincolnshire

IT WAS A PLEASURE to go to Lincolnshire in the spring. In the fields, tulip blooms stretched in ribbons of bright pink, red, yellow and white, from here to infinity.

Kate's Mum and Dad were held in high regard in the village, on account of the fact that they were not born in the village and not educated in the village school. Tony was the manager of the Horticultural Nursery in the village. The nursery had forty acres of heated glasshouses, banana ripening facilities, packing sheds and several farms attached. It was the largest employer in the area.

The part of Lincolnshire where my in-laws lived is known as Holland, on the east coast near The Wash. Reclaimed and drained marsh land has become fine, black, loamy soil, very rich and fertile. The main occupation is still arable farming. In those days it was an isolated place, most people had no reason to go there. It is now within commuting distance from London.

Windswept and largely treeless, save for the odd row of poplars planted as a windbreak, it is a place of wide, open skies, fresh air and hardy people. Face east in Lincolnshire and there are no real hills until the Ural Mountains in Russia. The wind from the east comes in straight from Siberia. Kate's parents lived in the middle of the village, in a large old farmhouse. The house had no central heating, and the doors and window frames were loose. In the winter, frost formed on the inside of the bedroom windows as well as outside. The big open log fires in the drawing room and the dining room were kept burning with sweet smelling applewood most of the time.

During a stay one winter, Tony would come into our bedroom and open the window. "You need some fresh air blowing in!" I invariably closed it as soon as he left, but he always came back and opened it again. "It's a lovely morning!" he'd say in his cheerful way as he pulled the sash window down again.

He was fond of military music and he tuned in every morning to a radio programme that seemed to specialise in brass band marches. The music permeated the house so we could hear it every morning, almost like a wake-up call.

In a telephone conversation he once said: 'Sat I've have got central heating now, it's made a *world* of difference. You can come over now, whatever the time of year, depth of winter even." He neglected to mention that his version of central heating was three electric storage heaters, one in the kitchen, one in the downstairs hall, and one in his own bedroom.

Kate always warned: "Before we go to see Mum and Dad, for goodness sake dress for the weather, thermal vest, long-johns, waist-coat, thick socks and tractor-tread boots, OK?" I did not listen to her advice, so I learnt the hard way.

One winter day Tony, Kate and I visited Henry's Shed, a veritable treasure trove of junk; heavy farm machinery, stuffed animals, wellington boots, Persian rugs and dolly tubs stood in every corner. Cracked tea sets, gas masks, costume jewellery and old clocks were piled onto shelves. Henry's Shed was deep in the heart of the fenlands, miles away from anywhere. All the wares were housed in barns with corrugated iron roofs and bare earthen floors. I bought a stuffed stag's head with horns and two large gun carriage wheels with solid brass hub caps, dating back possibly to the Crimean War.

It was an extremely cold day and I had worn my city shoes, no thermal underwear and a short donkey jacket. I

63

became so cold and stiff that I could not move. Back at The Chestnuts, I was hauled out of the car and into the kitchen. Kate and Dad thawed me out with my back against the storage heater, hot water bottles at my feet, and a large hot whisky-mac in my hand. This became a family joke, especially as I vowed not to visit Lincolnshire again during the winter months and especially to go nowhere near Henry's Shed.

In Tony's Horticultural Nursery, the packing shed was a sea of bright yellow daffodils, their fragrance overpowering, waiting to be loaded into wooden crates and transported to Covent Garden. Hyacinths, a fragrant cloud of blue, pink and white, guaranteed to bloom on Mother's Day, were boxed and ready to be sold in department stores and supermarkets up and down the country. They were the most popular choice of little customers, eager to delight their Mummy on Mothering Sunday.

I was fascinated with his nursery as he had an old fashioned but effective heating system, requiring coal fed boilers which produced steam that was carried in large pipes around the greenhouses. The boilers were housed in a large boiler house, at the back of the nursery. The boiler house had a concrete floor and brick walls. A mountain of coal was piled up outside. The boilers required an attendant, on duty in shifts, twenty-four hours a day and every day of the year, except in the height of summer, when the boilers were shut down and had an annual service. Tony was a very conscientious boss and visited the boiler men every day, especially at weekends and bank holidays; we even celebrated our family Firework Night there. He made a point of taking them a bottle of something on Christmas day. Kate told me "As a youngster I loved visiting the boiler men with Dad. They had a cosy office with a huge leather armchair, they had tea making equipment and a resident cat. When

64

they saw us coming, they'd get up from the armchair with "Allo! Now then Kathleen, what *you* up to?" She added: "I watched as they tucked *Playboy* magazine under the cushion and brought out an ancient copy of *Encyclopaedia Britannica*." I'd say: "Can I see the fire inside the boiler? Can I sit in your chair? Can I have a look at that big book?" "Yus, to all three" they'd say, and I'd marvel at the roaring fire in the boilers, be frightened of the pressure gauges on the outside of the boilers and sit in the armchair and thumb through the *Encyclopaedia*."

The nursery also had 'trickle irrigation' whereby each plant had its own water supply. A number of occasions, on walking in his nursery I was amazed with the results he achieved in producing plants from seeds. One of his tips, which I use when gardening, is that if you want a plant to flower, do not give water or feed. The plant will think it is going to die and produce the next generation.

As I mentioned, Holland, Lincolnshire is in a flat, sparsely populated county where most people are involved in agriculture and, during the winter when the land is too wet for ploughing, game and wild fowl shooting on the marshes is popular. There are many RAF bases in the flat lands of the fens and I have been a number of times to see air shows at Waddington and Scampton. Kate said: "Mum and Dad met on Scampton Air Base during the Second World War. Dad was an aircrew radio operator and had just returned from four years in the Western Desert in Egypt. Mum was a telephonist on Scampton's switchboard. The romance blossomed and after the war they got married.

Tony came with us once to Scampton's Air Show. He recalled his youthful flying days and he never lost the ability to translate anything into morse code. The highlight of the show was heralded by a low, steady rumble away in the distance. The rumble grew louder and suddenly overhead

65

there appeared a huge Lancaster Bomber, flanked by two Spitfires. The majestic flypast and the deep drone of the engines brought tears to Tony's eyes as he stood to attention.

During the second world war, Lincolnshire was known as Bomber County and the airbases there played a pivotal role during the conflict.

One of the most famous missions – 617 Squadron's Dam Buster raid in 1943 to bomb dams and disrupt industrial production in the Ruhr valley in Germany, flew from RAF Scampton. Of the 19 Lancaster Bombers that took part in the attacks carrying 133 crew, eight planes and 56 men were lost.

RAF Scampton is also home to the nine Red Arrows aerobatic team. But in 2022, when Scampton closes, they will move to RAF Waddington, also in Lincolnshire. We had the privilege to talk to some of the Red Arrows pilots. They told us they fly Hawk T Mark 1 aircraft, with a Rolls Royce Sidora engine. They fly between 6 and 11 feet apart at a top speed of 400mph. They experience -4G.

Kate herself clatters aloft occasionally in a small Cessna aircraft with an instructor by her side and I sit in the back with my video camera; she follows the river Humber to the coast, then turns round and comes back. "You OK back there, Sat?" she says. I usually reply: "I feel safer up here than I do with you on the M1!"

The little village of Quadring is on the A152, between Boston and Spalding. Boston, in the heart of the fens, is the town from which The Pilgrim Fathers set off across the Atlantic to America. Immigrants fleeing religious persecution, they landed in Massachusetts during the early 1600s and named their new American town *Boston*.

Spalding was home to the Tulip Festival that used to be held in May every year. Millions of tulips are grown and when they reach their peak, the heads are snapped off to create a bigger bulb. The tulip heads were used to make huge colourful floats, which paraded through the town. The festival attracted thousands of visitors.

Close friends of my parents-in-law had an acre or two of land in which they dug a lake. They bought exotic ducks, geese, hens, and a number of wallabies. They were keen on salmon fishing and made a trip to Scotland every year for the season. "You want to come with us Sat," they said, "We'll teach you how to cast your line." So, the next time they came over, my line casting skills over our clothes washing line were critically appraised. I'm happy to say that I have been successful due to their tutorials. I was able to catch a magnificent sixteen pounder when I went to Ireland on a flyfishing trip with friends some time ago. These same friends kindly gave us some of their chickens and ducks who became the beloved pets for our children.

Kate showed me the wild beauty of the fens; the big, big skies, featuring spectacular sunrises and sunsets; the skylarks that soar high into the air hovering above their nests; the *dykes* or canals, for drainage of the fenland and the marshes, stretching all the way to the sea; the truly wild undrained land on the other side of the sea walls.

The creeks here are tidal. It is essential to know the times of the tides if you venture onto the marshes. The tides vary with the time of year, but they also change daily. There's no more relaxing way to spend an afternoon than to go out on the salt flats and gather samphire, watch the wading birds and collect crabs; but, come evening, if you see a whirlpool of water in the creek then you know the tide has turned and you had better head for home, quick! Once the tide comes over the last sea wall, it will come in faster than you can run. Water flows into the creeks so quickly that in half an hour, where you stand will be under the sea for the next eight hours.

As I was driving home from Lincolnshire, early one morning, all around me the countryside's animal activity was on full display. Hares jumped on their hind legs in the fields, boxing with great gusto. I heard the calls of the pheasants and saw the gaudy males strutting their stuff to impress the females. But I was going home, to God's own county: Yorkshire is my home.

9. A Spiritual Journey

MY FAMILY follow a branch of Hinduism known as Arya Samaj, meaning "Noble Society." Members of Arya Samaj believe in one almighty Creator, as set out in the ancient texts of *The Vedas*. The Creator is the source of all knowledge, and members of Arya Sumaj are seekers after Truth and Knowledge. All acts in this life should be carried out after seeking the Truth, carried out with Knowledge, and guided by Love. The prime object of Arya Sumaj is to Do Good to the Whole World, the goodness of One is the goodness of All.

The founder of Arya Sumaj, Dayananda Saraswati, said: "There are undoubtedly many learned men among followers of every religion. Should they free themselves from Prejudice, accept the Universal Truths (that is, those truths that are to be found alike in all Religions and are of Universal Application), reject all things in which the various religions differ, and if they treat each other Lovingly, it will be greatly to the Advantage of the World."

The practice of helping our fellow human beings has pervaded our family life to this present day. Kate and our children go along with this philosophy. My parents were so proud to offer my services to the sick and disabled. Our family house in India had recently been connected to the telephone system so my mother would now phone the temple, instead of making a visit, and say: "My son, who is a doctor in England, is coming next week. If you would like to organise a clinic, he will see as many sick as he can."

Medical consultations cost money to all but the very poor in India, so she was offering a very valuable service. When I worked at Barnsley Hospital, they knew I provided these consultations, and on one occasion a medical representative phoned the day before Kate and I were to go to India, saying: "Can I pop over? I've got £6,000 worth of anti-TB and anti-Leprosy drugs here that have *just* gone out of date!"

He called and delivered six cardboard boxes. So we took medicines to India that could no longer be used in the United Kingdom.

The lane leading to my parents' house is one-car wide, so taxis prefer to drop off at the top of the lane. The house is at the end of a small cul-de-sac of about ten houses. Life in the cul-de-sac is lived communally and everyone knows their neighbours' comings and goings. As our taxi drew up, everyone left their chores and came out to lean on their garden gate.

Kate and I acknowledged the reception committee as we wheeled our baggage along the dust lane. All eyes followed us as we were, in effect, guests of the street. My mother, standing at the end of the narrow lane, had been waiting for us since dawn. Once the neighbours had seen Kate and me drop down to touch my parents' feet in greeting, they would return to where they had left off, although not before making a mental note to visit our house as soon as possible.

Thus, our arrival soon reached the ears of the temple and on the following day, they rang. "Welcome Home!" they would greet me; and, after the usual enquiries after our health and the journey, they would request: "Can you come tomorrow?" My reply was always "Yes." "Can you come at six?" My reply was again: "Yes" "See you tomorrow *morning* then!"

We had a steady stream of patients for ten hours, but it seemed like ten minutes. When we had finally seen the last patient and as we packed up, Kate said: "Well, we've seen all ages, from tiny babies to the very elderly, and every age in between."

Yes," I replied, "carried on stretchers, or come here by walking, rickshaw or bicycle, and the whole of the local orphanage and school checked over too."

Some patients I diagnosed and could help, as I gave out my free medicines. But some were beyond help, so I gave painkillers. One, I remember, came crippled with polio. Three drops of vaccine on a sugar cube would have spared her a lifetime with a twisted spine and unequal legs. Then some would come coughing and emaciated, and I knew the TB drugs would have been a life- saver for them if only they had been caught earlier.

Once we visited Mother Teresa's Hospital for the Dying and Destitute. There we met a woman of unknown age. She had been either lost or abandoned in the jungle as a child and had probably survived on berries, fruits, roots and insects. Eventually she was found crawling around the outskirts of a village. She was wild and could neither walk nor talk. She grunted and snorted and refused to enter a house or sleep on a bed. No one knew where she had come from, so she was brought to Mother Teresa's Hospital in Meerut. Here the nuns tenderly cared for her. They arranged that she sleep outside, as she had been used to, but they kept her in the safety of the hospital courtyard. They brought her food and water in bowls, as she ate from the floor.

When we met her, she had been bathed and shampooed and her matted hair had been cut short. She lay on a mattress on the floor with her food and water bowls beside her. We had taken our youngest daughter Jane, about 18 months old, with us, and the woman was fascinated with her. She played with Jane, while they grunted and gurgled at each other. In all the world, all she wanted now was lots of cuddles so whilst Jane chuckled and patted her face, the woman cradled her in her arms. She then went back to crawling around the courtyard.

Inside the hospital, we were beckoned to his bedside by the most skeletal man I had ever seen. His yellow face was like tissue paper and his long thin arms stretched out to hold Jane. We placed her in his embrace. He beamed the most angelic and peaceful smile and said: "Hello, Baby" in English. She sat on his coverlet while he held her tiny hand. We picked her up again as he sighed and lay back on his pillow, exhausted. We put a donation in an envelope and left.

One of my regular patients was a girl who was profoundly deaf in both ears; she could hear nothing, and so could not speak properly either. She had visited me for seventeen years, every time I came on a visit to see my parents.

We all knew that the operation that would restore her hearing, known as a Cochlear Implant, was not available in India at that time. Her family could not afford the trip to the UK or America for the operation. The post-operative back-up after these implants is considerable and their funds would certainly not have covered an extended stay abroad.

At twenty-three years old, time was slipping by. I explained that, once again, I had not brought a cure for her. In her frustration, she lashed out. "You *said* there is a cure for me!" she mouthed awkwardly. "If you got an operation for me," she prodded me angrily in the chest, "I could get married and have a lovely life!" She was 23 years old, and time was slipping by. Marriage with a handicap is not normally acceptable in India. These implants are readily done now in India, at a price, but too late for her.

I had friends in school and college from differing faiths and communities, but religion was never an issue. I was surrounded by Christians, Sikhs, Muslims, Buddhists, and other Hindu sects such as Jains and Parsis. Birth, life, and rebirth (re-incarnation or life after death) was one belief we all had in common. Most believed in one God. Many representations of the one God are believed by mainstream Hindus. Most instantly recognisable are Sikhs, in turbans and beards. Theirs is the newest sect, begun over 500 years ago by Guru Nanak. A meal will always be provided at a Gurdwara, a Sikh Temple.

Muslim girls were in my college class. They travelled to school wearing a burka, a long flowing robe covering the body, head and half of the face but they removed it in the classroom. I was interested in all religions and had attended church services and Sikh festivals. Hindus and Sikhs are more than willing to participate in everyone's feast days and festivals.

"Let's go and see what Christmas is like in Sardhana!" said one of my friends during our winter school break. Sardhana is a small town fifteen miles north of my hometown of Meerut. Sardhana, although only a small town, has a large Roman Catholic Cathedral, the Sacred Heart Boys' School, a Centre for Voluntary Work, and a Presbytery. It was run by an Italian order. We arrived by bus. People from near and far and of all faiths spilled out of the many buses to join in the festivities and attend the Christmas and Easter Services.

We celebrated the Hindu festivals of Holi, Deshera and Diwali. Holi is the Hindu equivalent of Easter; Dussehra could be likened to Bonfire Night. And Diwali, the festival of light, is like Christmas.

After spending a year serving in hospitals in Delhi, I arrived in London for post-graduation studies. My second job in Worcester gave me an opportunity to experience an English town with a magnificent Cathedral. I attended Christmas celebrations with friends from the hospital. During a discussion in the ward sister's office, I gathered Christians have beliefs and sacraments performed in the ward for patients who are very ill. After working in Cambridge and Plymouth, I had landed my Registrar job in Nottingham. There is a large Roman Catholic Cathedral near the hospital and Catholic Priests visited the wards and the Intensive Care department on a regular basis. The medical staff's efforts were directed towards keeping the patient comfortable and alive, and Priests were concerned with the patient's peace of mind.

To marry Kate, I agreed to bring up any children we might have in the Roman Catholic faith. After our marriage, we lived in a little apartment near the hospital in Stoke-on-Trent. Sometimes I attended Sunday morning Mass with Kate. "I'm under instruction," I announced as Kate cooked the supper one evening. She was non-committal with her "Oh, that's good" reply. Inwardly, she told herself: "It won't last, so don't raise your hopes, Kate!"

It was very interesting to discuss the Catholic viewpoint with our very well-read and knowledgeable Priest. He understood my confusion about the Virgin birth, which he did try to explain to me – but without much success.

We moved to Birmingham where our first child was born. I continued my instructions in the Faith, in our new parish. We again returned to Stoke-on-Trent, this time I worked at The Infirmary, but we attended the same church as before. I enrolled for instruction again.

"Aah, Dr Mehta, you're back again! Not taken the plunge yet?" said the astonished parish priest, as I embarked on a third year of discussion. After a particularly lengthy conversation with the priest, I was still not sure about a

74

Virgin birth, so in the end he said: "It's a miracle, Sat, and you either accept it or you don't, that's why it's called *faith!*" "OK," I said, "I accept it!" and I was welcomed into the church with a glass of whisky.

We are a family of regular churchgoers, involved in social activities, voluntary work, and fundraising for charities. My local church in Wakefield is very friendly and vibrant, involved in good work both locally and overseas.

We have a charity unique to our parish called The Suzy Fund. It was started by our friends Brian and Lynne, when they saw a photo of a little girl in Ethiopia, dying of starvation and thrown away on a rubbish dump. They named her Suzy.

Brian owned a business and in 1975 he asked his employees to donate 10p a week to his Suzy Fund. Brian and Lynne brought the fundraising to our church too. Over the years, we have done many fund-raising activities at different houses; barbecues, plant sales, musical functions and fun runs.

The Suzy charity up till now has raised nearly a million pounds.

The charity has no expenses since all the fund-raising is done by volunteers. A hundred per cent of the money raised goes to our projects in developing countries. One of our projects involved running a clean water supply to a village in Africa. Brian himself went to see, at his own expense, how the initiative had improved the life there.

He sat down with the Village Chief. "Well," said Brian, "How's life, now you have a clean water tap to every household in the village?"

The Chief grinned. "Terrible!" he replied, "all the women are depressed!" He chuckled: "They're not going

75

down to the river any more, so no gossiping on the riverbank!"

The Suzy Fund has financed vaccinations, water pumps and soup kitchens, from Romania to Rwanda, and all from the compassion, tireless enthusiasm and drive of one couple's love for our fellow human beings.

Whether you call it Christian or Hindu, the result is what matters.

10. The Midlands

TO GAIN EXPERIENCE, junior doctors move jobs every six months. This often means moving from hospital to hospital and town to town. In 1971, we moved from Stoke upon Trent to Birmingham and 1972 saw me return to Stoke with promotion; in 1974 I was promoted again and worked in Birmingham and Coventry.

During my spell in the Potteries, I gained experience in General Surgery covering conditions of the abdomen and bowel; Vascular surgery, dealing with conditions of the blood vessels; Thoracic surgery, dealing with conditions involving the respiratory system and chest; and finally, Neurosurgery, dealing with conditions involving the nerves, spinal cord and brain. They were all very busy jobs, and I learnt a great deal.

Since then, if a patient comes to me describing a list of seemingly unrelated symptoms, my experience in other specialities has been helpful in diagnosis. The day is fast approaching when robots will perform operations, but listening to the patient's symptoms, observing the patient's bodily signs, and interpreting the right tests, is where human experience counts.

I once had a patient who consulted me about her voice loss, sore throat, and swollen abdomen She said her throat had never felt right since an exploratory gynaecological operation six months previously. Under anaesthesia I could find nothing wrong with her throat. She had told me of her extreme fatigue, loss of weight and swollen abdomen. There was indeed something wrong with her. I noticed multiple small reddish lumps on her upper chest. I biopsied two and sent them to the laboratory for analysis. She went home that evening and we waited for the laboratory result. Two days later I had the unhappy responsibility to call her and her husband to come and see me.

The result of the biopsy was devastating. Malignant cells, found in the laboratory sample, showed cells originating from an Ovarian Cancer. I said they must urgently consult her gynaecologist again and suggested that a scan of her abdomen and pelvis would reveal the extent of the malignancy.

Sadly, her cancer had become inoperable and terminal. I continued to visit her at home and made sure she was pain-free until she died. How incongruous, I thought, that piecing a jigsaw together, or following a trail like a detective, observing the whole patient, should lead from a sore throat to a distant inoperable cancer.

Paediatricians – baby and child specialists – are very good at interpretation and "child speak." So, when the little patient says: "I've got a headache," the specialist says: "Where is the headache?" knowing full well the "headache" could be anywhere. "It's right here" says the child and points to the abdomen.

The Neuro-surgical job was very busy. The Consultant was a gifted surgeon and his whole team worked hard. Patients came from near and far to see him. Operating lists started earlier than anyone else's and finished after most surgical teams had packed up and gone home. Lunch breaks were often missed completely and operations rolled on into the evening. After the last patient left the theatre, there would then be a ward round to check up on all the other patients. After that, a visit to Intensive Care, to see the newly operated. The Neuro-surgical Consultant worked hard, and he played hard too.

One day, Kate and I were invited to a party at his home. That evening the operating list finished late, and the team ate nothing the whole day. After finishing the ward round, I went home, had a shower, a quick change of clothes and off we went to the house party.

Most of the department staff were there and many other guests besides. The neurosurgeon brewed his own beer and made wine too. He often described wine he had made from the most wonderful and strange fruits and vegetables, even nettles. We knew the home-made beer and wine would be flowing at the party and sure enough: "Ah! Sat! Kate!" my Consultant exclaimed as he opened the door to us, "Welcome! Come in, we are all here now, go to the lounge. Before you do, get a pint of my classic beer or a big glass of my new sparkling elderflower wine from the kitchen."

I was very thirsty and hungry, as I had missed my lunch and tea, nothing to eat since breakfast. I downed the pint straight away and almost immediately I had a second pint put in my hand. We were having a great time, chatting with our friends and other guests, and it certainly was a party that went with a swing.

Before I knew it, I had drunk my third pint and nibbled on the snacks that were handed round. The full buffet still lay in splendour on the dining room table and was yet to be served. I must have been on my fourth homebrew pint by now and was feeling very merry. I was unsteady on my feet and I began to slur my speech.

My Consultant, a fitness enthusiast, kept his gym equipment in the sitting room. Some of the guests were quite intrigued by it. I cannot remember, but I must have wandered towards the equipment and started trying it out. I began showing the gathering crowd of guests how to use every gadget, particularly a roller that rolled along on the floor. Kate was on the other side of room, saw the gathering throng and heard that someone was doing a demonstration of the gym equipment. She came across and – to her utter horror – saw me rolling back and forth on the floor. "This is how you use it, Sir," I bellowed to my Consultant.

With the help of a colleague who shared duties with me, Kate bundled me into the back of our car, and we arrived back home. I had been so drunk I could not remember that my work colleague had chuckled: "I'll take the head end and you take his feet, Kate." And I was carried down the garden path, through the front door and dumped fully clothed on our bed.

The following morning, the effect of my over-indulgence had receded, except for a thumping headache and intense nausea. I decided to go to the department, and I apologised to my Colleagues and other staff for being drunk the previous night.

"Don't worry," they said, "somebody should have warned you! We've come across his homebrew before – nobody knows the percentage of alcohol, least of all the brewer!" They did, however, relate to me in detail how I instructed the Consultant in the use of his own gym equipment.

My Consultant was, as usual, busy in theatre, on the second case already, and I was supposed to have been there to assist. "I'm sorry about last night," I eventually stammered.

"I'm surprised you're here at all," he laughed. "Listen, you go home, I can manage here. Back to bed, Sat."

It was about 9 pm one winter's night and I was two hours into my all-night shift at Birmingham's GP Deputising Service, covering the rough, poor areas that night. A colleague on the same shift, but covering the better-off, leafy suburban lanes at the other side of the city, rang me for some advice. He had been called by the anxious parents of a little girl. On getting her ready for bed, they were horrified to see a large creamy white tissue dangling from her anus. My colleague arrived at the house and examined the little patient. He suspected her lower bowel had prolapsed and squeezed out through her anus. This would mean admittance to hospital and an operation to place it back inside the body.

He decided to ask me for a second opinion. I arrived half an hour later, pulled on a pair of rubber gloves and examined the child. She had a persistent cough but otherwise was well. "Have you been abroad, lately, on holiday perhaps?" I asked.

The father replied: "Well, we had two weeks in south east Asia last month, but we were never ill with anything. We were really careful."

"Yes," said the mother, "Especially with little Emily here. She was fine, never ill with a thing apart from coughing bouts!"

"Well," I said, "What I've found will surprise you then, but it's good news and easily cured." I gently pulled the creamy white "tissue" free – and there, in my hand, lay a large wriggling round worm, the size of my middle finger. I kept pulling out more worms until no more appeared. The parents gasped and the mother turned away in disgust.

"You see," I said, "Sadly, in my part of the world these worms, and many other types are not uncommon. I've come across these many times. We don't need the hospital, but we are writing a letter to your doctor, who will prescribe tablets and arrange a stool test to confirm worm eggs."

My colleague said: "This is the first time I have ever seen a round worm! Thank you!" We handed the letter over and I left to hurry back to my own patch of Birmingham.

11. Country Life

IN 1976, we were looking to buy a house within an eight-mile radius of the hospital, as I had a Senior Registrar post now and so did not have to live within five minutes of the place.

Kate, being a country girl, was relieved to get out of Birmingham "Let's look for a house in the countryside!" she said. We found Barlaston village, home to the Wedgwood factory, with a house for sale on the end of a row, near open fields. The house was within walking distance of the canal, the railway station and six miles from the hospital. We had already sold our house in Birmingham and were able to complete the contract in six weeks.

The new house was open-plan sixties style, but with a real fireplace which also had a back boiler to heat water. There were silver birch trees in the front garden; and to the back of the house was a lawn, a greenhouse, a vegetable patch and a small orchard.

That summer was the hottest for many years. Tar melted on the roads, moors and heathland smouldered and burst into flame, rivers dried up and water was rationed. Our new neighbours were friendly and knowledgeable gardeners with many years' experience. I learned from them to grow vegetables and fruits. My bedtime reading was *Be Your Own Garden Expert* and *The Vegetable Plotter*. To our amazement, with the extra hot weather, we were able to grow lettuce, radish, cabbage, cauliflower, beetroot, peas, broad beans and other vegetables; and to top that, we were able to grow corn on the cob, melon, chillies and aubergines in the greenhouse.

The house was near the railway line and hearing the trains go by brought back childhood memories of my Dad's working on coal wagons in the shunting yard. A short walk took us to the village green, the canal, a woodland walk and the small railway station. We could travel by boat to nearby places, passing through tranquil and wonderful scenery. There were ducks, moor hens and jumping trout in the canal.

We had two children at that time: Louise and Paul. Louise started at the Convent School in the nearby town of Stone. The school was next to the church we attended.

The parish priest was Father O'Leary who became a personal friend. He often visited to discuss cars, gardening and sport. He would stay to have a bite to eat with me: as the working hours of both of us were irregular, he could be sure I would not be home for my evening meal before 9pm, so he could call by and we'd sit, one each side of the fire, with trays on our laps.

One evening he visited and stayed to have a meal with me, as Kate had eaten earlier with the children. Apart from the normal curry, rice and chapattis, Kate put a large dish of chilli pickle on the trays. Before I could stop him, Father finished his whole dish of pickle. "Very tasty, that sure was very tasty, Kathleen!" he said, wiping his brow. The following morning, he said Mass as usual. He must have had a very strong stomach.

Father occasionally called me to ask if I would call at the Convent to see one of the Sisters with an ear, nose or throat complaint, and he would meet me there. We would exit the Convent by way of a little winding path through the Convent Cemetery. "D'you need any cuttings for the garden?" he would enquire "All my best cuttings come from cemeteries."

During a visit to Cannock Chase one day, I suggested to Kate that I could teach her to drive off-road, in the woods, "But you'd have to mind the trees." I warned.

This was a mistake. I think we did fall out temporarily and decided that she should have proper driving lessons from a qualified instructor. At that time, we owned an old Vauxhall Viva car. It was a good car except, no matter how hard we pressed the pedal, it would not accelerate.

Stupidly, we decided to have a holiday exploring the hills and valleys of Wales. The car chugged along but refused to scale anything more than a slight incline, so we would push it uphill, then freewheel down the other side. I remember the days when motoring demanded more of a pioneering spirit, broken down cars on the roadside, drivers' legs visible from under the chassis, or the bonnet up and a driver with sleeves rolled up to the elbow and black grease everywhere. There was camaraderie amongst us motorists then, a comradeship, you could even say a companionship, and a mechanical champion would come along at any moment and say: "If I can't fix it, I'll get you to the nearest garage, mate."

12. Children

OUR FIRST CHILD Louise was born in Birmingham in 1971. We treated her like the most delicate china, afraid she might break at any moment, until we had the advice of a splendid lady with a family of six. "A warm heart and a firm confident hand are what babies like," she said, patting Louise's bottom very firmly so our little baby bounced up and down.

Louise is warm and outgoing, always involved in whatever excitement is going on. When she was small, we had to have eyes in the back of our heads. She was two years old when one cold and frosty morning, wearing only her little vest, she bolted out the front door and toddled away down the hill, her tiny bare bottom glinting in the morning sunshine. Happily, she ran straight into the arms of our milkman who scooped her up and put her on his milk float. He delivered her to our door, along with three pints of milk.

Once again, off on her travels, aged four, she went missing one Saturday morning. Neighbours to the rescue this time. The two teenage sons of a serving police officer burst out of their garden gate and joined the search, when they heard Kate bellowing "Louise, where are you!" on the street.

"We'll call the station and see if Dad can come with his police-dog, if we don't find her in half an hour! We'll need an unwashed item of her clothes." They dashed up the street towards Birmingham's main arterial road into the city. Kate spent an agonising twenty minutes, pacing back and forth in front of the phone. When the boys re-appeared, a happy Louise was bouncing on their shoulders. "Oh! Thank you, thank you! Where did you find her?"

They grinned "We don't know how she crossed the road, but she was knocking on the playschool door."

"Oh, thank you!!" was all Kate could stammer at that moment. But later, Louise and Kate delivered a big homemade chocolate cake and a thank you card to the boys' house.

Louise's curiosity sometimes led to dire consequences. She opened the supposedly "child-proof" top of a sealed tub of junior aspirins and swallowed the lot. Kate noticed the open tub and immediately we took her to the Children's Hospital where she had a stomach washout and was admitted overnight.

In the last year at school, a Leaver's Ball was held. Louise had a beautiful white taffeta dress made. To go with this, she had seen some silver and diamante, peep-toed, stiletto-heeled shoes. "No, choose something else," Kate said, "too high, too narrow and *far* too expensive!"

But Louise had set her heart on them. The following day, at school lunchtime, she took a train to Leeds and purchased the shoes. Unfortunately, that day luck was not on her side. She boarded the return train: not only was it delayed by 20 minutes but she sat in stunned silence opposite the thunderous face of her teacher!

That afternoon we received a call from the Headmistress. Kate wearily said: "I'm on my way, shall I come to your office?" So Louise learnt the error of her ways from both Kate and the Headmistress, in no uncertain terms.

Louise was a keen footballer and joined her brother and his friends in many a game on the back lawn. The boys gave her no quarter as her tackling was legendary. At school she enjoyed Classics and English but Dancing was where she positively shone with her effortlessly graceful style.

Always one to have-a-go, she joined the Territorial Army. No fancy shoes or make-up here! Hair scraped back in a bun and uniform belted in the middle, she went for The Initial Training Camp. It was held on the vast and windswept

North York Moors. It rained the whole weekend. They pitched the tents, groundsheet first, so it was thoroughly soaked by the time they put up the flysheet,

"They'll have to learn the hard way," thought the Sergeant. Louise agreed to cook. She stirred the porridge over an open fire, as if she were mixing cement, the raindrops ran off her nose and the porridge gained a salty and smoky flavour. She brought some home for us to try but none of us had a stomach strong enough to eat more than a teaspoonful.

The training weekend included an obstacle course, crawling through thick mud and wet bracken. As she scrambled up and over high walls, someone's big hand would descend to haul her over the top, with a "Give us your hand, you wimp!" That evening the Sergeant prodded her awake when she fell asleep during a security video, shouting: "OI, YOU, WAKE UP!!"

On the last night, totally unannounced, Princess Anne, the TA Colonel-in-Chief, just walked into the hut, totally unannounced, poured herself a cup of coffee and sat down for a chat. Louise loved the camaraderie of the company and enthused when she came home: "By the end of that training we'd have trusted each other with our lives, we've been through *so much* together!" When she went to university in London, she left the TA but cherishes the memories of the friends she met.

When Louise was 16 she fell in love. The relationship was intense for ones so young. They were together all day, and in touch by walkie-talkie radio and stones on the bedroom window at night. He was welcomed into our house and really became part of the family, so frequent a caller was he. The whole neighbourhood must have viewed them as a modern-day Romeo and Juliet.

One spring, Kate and I were in India with our two

youngest children. The two eldest had not wanted to come: "We are busy at school," they said, "see if Grandfather will come over to look after us." So, Grandfather Tony came; but under his new home management, the rules suddenly changed. The boyfriend was stopped from bounding straight upstairs, as Grandfather boomed: "Excuse me, young man, you may wait for Louise in the drawing *rhum*." He added: "I'll let her know you're here." As they were going through the front door, Grandfather further issued his code of conduct, "I'd like you to escort Louise back here by 10pm, not a minute later! "

During her gap year, Louise went to America to spend time at the Coca-Cola Young People's Training Camp. There she taught English Language, Grammar and Dance.

Later she visited Israel and stayed in a Kibbutz. She went to university in London and had a very successful career in IT Recruitment. She was invited by her employer to work in their Sydney branch and thus she left England and settled in Australia. She is now married with a daughter of her own.

Paul is our second child, born in Stoke-on-Trent in 1973. The school to which he went is on the outskirts of Wakefield and was, at that time, all boys and partly boarding. He was quiet and shy when he started, but the school had a wonderful can-do attitude, a robust sport and outdoor pursuit programme and a great set of boys and staff. So, he gradually gained knowledge, confidence, and a great sense of humour.

"Mehta, you're Indian, aren't you?" the sports master enquired.

Paul replied, "*Dad* is, Sir!"

"That's near enough, you're in the cricket team!" And so, Paul played cricket for the school.

He was also in the cross-country team. One rainy Saturday morning, a few of the cross-country team set off for a run up the long hill past the glue factory on the aptly named Stinkhouse Lane. The rain began to pelt down, and a kind lady stopped to offer a lift to the bedraggled group. Hot and steamy, they piled into her car, dripping mud everywhere and fogging the windows "Where to, boys?" she brightly enquired.

"This is absolutely *very* kind of you, *amazing*, really, really *great*," the boys enthused as they realised that it was none other than their Headmaster's wife at the wheel, "If you could just drop us somewhere near the school further up *outside* the school gates, please?"

"Well, that's funny," she chuckled, "I'm going there myself!" Luckily, she failed to see the coincidence.

He still enjoys running for charity to this day. He had the temerity to beat his headmaster at golf and is a keen tennis and squash player and was in the school teams. Paul's school was known for its sporting excellence, well-mannered boys, and charitable galas; the masters also worked hard on the academic achievement side of things too.

Paul would have been in his early teens when one day Kate took a phone call. "Neville Johnson, Bespoke Furniture here," said the bright voice on the end of the line "Could I speak to Mr Paul Mehta please?"

Kate said: "Ah, you mean Mr *Sat* Mehta."

"No," insisted the other, "it says Mr *Paul* Mehta here."

"Could I ask in what connection?" Kate enquired.

"Tell him it's about the lighting for his new swimming pool."

"No, really?" said Kate.

"Yes," added the caller, "And I've got the quote for the fitted office furniture too."

"Right!" said Kate, "I'll just call him from his *homework.*"

It was decided a hockey team should be formed, and Paul signed up. On the next Mothers' keep-fit evening class Kate attended at the school, she was talking to the Headmaster's wife. "The boys are looking to challenge another side at hockey," said the lady, "We don't have enough here to make up the numbers.

Kate chuckled "I'm sure the Girls' High School would be willing to give them a game. Shall I ask them? I've got three girls there." And so, it was arranged.

The day came and the boys were ready for an easy game. The girls' minibus drew up and their elite players ran onto the battlefield. Paul arrived home that evening looking the worse for wear. "Game go alright, dear?" enquired Kate, as Paul trailed mud and grass upstairs.

"Good Grief!!" Paul shouted over his shoulder, "They were like a load of wild animals! They got off the bus, badges sewn all the way down their shorts, sweatbands round their heads!" He rubbed his shins, "I don't think we'll ask them for a re-match," he said, "Anyway we didn't want to tackle 'em, they're girls – I think." He never told us what the score was.

Paul had a great set of friends, and in the last year of school they arranged a summer holiday on the Greek island of Corfu to celebrate their A level results. They decided it would be sensible to have soft drinks for the first day, until they knew where their accommodation was and how to get there. But evening came, they went out, and that resolve was forgotten. A few drinks led to a few more. At the end of the night, some managed to stagger to their hotel accommodation, but Paul lay down on the beach to ease the effects of Greek Sangria and English beer.

He curled up under the sea wall and went to sleep.

During the night, a tip-up truck piled high with squashed and rotting vegetables collected from the market, dumped its load over the sea wall and onto the sleeping Paul, but he slumbered on. The sun rose and the temperature climbed, the vegetables began to ferment. Three local elderly ladies finished their morning walk and sat down on the beach, gazing out to sea. Suddenly they were startled by a loud yawn behind them. Paul rose like a phoenix from its ashes, scattering squashed tomatoes and fermenting grapes in his wake. He was steaming and stinking, a cabbage leaf on his head slowly turning to green liquid as the ladies screamed and scrambled to their feet. They made off down the beach and Paul squelched back to the hotel.

During a family holiday in Barbados, Paul decided to ignore the *Safe Bathing* sign directly opposite our hotel and go down to the rocky shore and swim from there. Presently we were aware of a crowd of tourists gathering on the beach and agonised moans coming from the depths of the growing throng. It was Paul, rolling on the sand and waving his foot in the air. The tourists stood around helplessly, but the locals had seen it all before. A big motherly waitress from the hotel announced: "It's Sea Urchins, e's stood on Sea Urchins, an' what we need is some *pee*, we need some pee from someone!" No one moved.

We took our youngest child Jane to the ladies' toilet, and she obliged. The liquid was poured on the Sea Urchin spines stuck in Paul's foot, but to no avail. Then a local lad sauntered up and chuckled "Hot wax! I've got some hot wax!" and he helpfully lit a match and dripped hot candle wax onto the foot. We gathered that tourists regularly disregard the warning notices, and the locals are only too delighted to rush to their aid. We discovered first aid treatments involved the application of heat and/or ammonia administered as quickly as possible, usually right there on the beach. "Thank goodness you didn't sit on it," smirked Louise, "or your swim trunks would have been down, and hot wax would have dripped on your bum!"

When we moved to Wakefield, my father-in-law joked: "You know the old saying, Sat? New house, new baby!" And, after a seven-year gap, Kate's news that a baby was on the way came as a lovely surprise. Come to think of it, it worked the same for the house extension we built two years later!

Clare was born in the spring of 1979 and spent the first few months of her life staring up through the drooping fronds of our big green willow tree, gently swaying above her pram, and listening to birdsong in the trees and frogs croaking in the pond. This must have endowed her with her love of nature.

"I'm going to fetch eggs," she would say, as she toddled off down the garden path to the chicken coop in the orchard; there she would put her hand into the warm straw where our six hens laid their eggs. She remembers being very upset and cross with herself when, not having hands big enough to carry all the eggs, she put two in each pocket of her dress – but by the time she had made it all the way up to the house again, the eggs had cracked and the yolk ran in a gluey yellow stream down her legs and into her shoes.

When Clare was older, Kate often said: "Come in, it's getting dark" as Clare disappeared out the back door at dusk to lie beside the pond and listen to the chorus of croaking frogs.

Clare sent the little amount of pocket money she had to St Tiggywinkles Hospital for Sick and Injured Hedgehogs. She is fascinated by the natural world and during her childhood variously owned and cared for, two Mallard ducks, Donald, and Daisy; two budgerigars, Pepe, and Ollie; and two guinea pigs. She also helped her younger

92

sister Jane look after her hen Milly, the Aylesbury ducks, the goat, the two cats and the two rabbits. Clare's pets lived in luxury, having the run of her bedroom: indeed, Pepe and Ollie flew around her room as if they owned the place, pecking at the wallpaper, perching on the arm of her spectacles or combing through her hair with their beaks whilst she sat at her homework; and her guinea pigs squeaked in delight at being fed tasty morsels on the sunlit patch of floor underneath her desk; even the ducks were invited into the kitchen when the coast was clear and Kate and I were not at home.

If we could not find Clare by the pond or in the orchard, she would be curled up in a sunny spot engrossed in a book. Kate took her to the library twice a week, where she borrowed the maximum six books. Academic work at school came easily to her and she won scholarships all the way through junior and senior school. Clare took five A level subjects and passed with A star in all of them.

Paul was so impressed with Clare's academic excellence that he put her name up for the Mensa test when she was fifteen; she passed with the high-scoring mark of 162.

When she was about ten, Clare went, along with the rest of her class, on a PGL holiday (I'm told it stands for Parents Get Lost). And, although Kate went along as the group nurse, it was just as well the other mothers did not see their little darlings covered in mud and swinging over a stream on the end of a rope, or abseiling up a wall two storeys high. Archery, assault course, horse riding, quad biking and cycling skills filled their days; and at the end, a farewell disco.

Louise, Clare and Jane went to an all-girls school, so a disco with real live boys was something not to be missed; the girls felt the disco was a great success although the lads' chat-up lines lacked a little finesse, "D'ya fancy me then?" or "Oi, d'ya wanna dance wi' me?" But it seemed what the boys lacked in the finer points of masculine charm they made up for in energetic and inventive dance steps.

Clare decided to take a gap year before embarking on her university course, so she went on an expedition to Nepal, travelled through Chile, New Zealand, and Australia. A project in Hawaii with dolphins came next; and then she joined a coral reef conservation project on a remote and uninhabited Philippine island, where she stayed for two months. She scuba-dived day and night, with cave dives and night dives amongst the bioluminescent phytoplankton, that glow like thousands of tiny stars in the dark night sea. "I don't need my hair anymore, so I'm sending it home. It's rotting with sea water anyway" read the note that accompanied her beautiful long hair, wrapped up in a brown paper parcel when it arrived through our letter box one day. She had shaved her head.

During her medical degree at Imperial College in London, she chose to go to Belize and Ecuador for three months experience. "Is that gun shots I hear?" asked Kate, during a telephone conversation with her. "Yes, I'm in a phone box on the street," Clare went on calmly," It's a bit of a volatile place here. I had a patient today who came with a deep laceration in his head, and all he did was walk across his neighbour's garden!"

Jane, our youngest child, joined Clare on her travels in Mexico and arrived there on The Day of the Dead. The nation were honouring their ancestors, remembering dead relations and friends. Little market stalls sold paper skulls, face masks, plastic skeletons, and shrunken heads. The bakers' shops sold bread in the shape of corpses, some even had fake hair attached to their crusty heads.

Families brought picnic lunches and sat around the graves of their loved ones in the cemetery, enjoying all the deceased had enjoyed when alive. Children played around the gravestones whilst their grandmothers decorated the grave with framed photographs, candles, and flowers.

Later that week, Kate was woken at 3am by the ping of a text message on her phone. It was from Clare and it read: "Help! Jane crossed border through jungle from Guatemala to Mexico. Have met up but need medical advice. No real pharmacies so can't get drugs or dressings. She is covered with mosquito bites. Has open sores on ankles, wore scuba-diving fins two sizes too big. Bleeding, left ear drum from scuba-dive descent too quick."

Kate roused me from sleep in panic and we had to think hard what to advise when access to medical supplies is non-existent. Eventually I said, "Text this: 1. Tear off petticoat, blouse or anything clean cotton and rub same with garlic. 2. Put two drops of clean oil in Jane's ear (cooking oil will do) then plug ear with garlic treated cotton. DO NOT get ear wet, NO swimming until healed. 3. Rub her all over with garlic. 4. Both of you take up cigar smoking."

Kate looked up at this last suggestion. "To keep mosquitos away," I grinned.

Clare and Jane found that two young girls travelling unaccompanied in South America brought unwanted male attention, so they devised a plan. Clare wore her baggiest dungarees and Doc Marten boots, and her crew cut hair completed the look. Jane discarded her bra, wore a rainbow tee shirt and tied her hair in a bandana. They looked the part, especially if they held hands, and I'm sure the garlic helped too.

At one point, the girls decided they would like to try a traditional meal. The waiter brought two roast guinea pigs with their little paws still attached, accompanied by roast potatoes and vegetables. History does not record what happened next.

Jane was born in February 1981. Kate was totally alone in the hospital when Jane arrived. We do not know the time of her birth, but Kate recalls the birds began to sing outside the frosted glass of the ground floor window.

Jane was cute and small, and her sisters Louise and Clare and her brother Paul wanted to look after her. Paul, however, had *really* wanted a baby brother, so, on the principle that wishing makes dreams come true, he told his teacher the good news, but changed the facts a little. So, Kate was surprised to see, written large on the whiteboard in Paul's classroom: "Mehta's family have a new baby. It is a boy, and his name is John." So, Jane's nickname was Jonty from that day forth.

Jane has always had a wonderful way with people, there to help whenever and whatever the need, right from childhood. She would have been about seven when one of her school friends confided that her brother came into her room each night and put a pillow over her face. Poor Jane agonised over her friend's imminent murder, so she decided to ask the teacher for help in preventing it.

Her fears were calmed when the teacher said she would keep a very close eye on the situation: but, as the victim turned up for school every morning, and as her friend seemed unperturbed by her nightly ordeals, Jane need not lose any more sleep. "Mrs Mehta, don't *ever* let your daughter become a social worker, will you!" the teacher said to Kate, "The worry would kill her!"

Our three elder children's bedrooms were usually in a state of complete disarray. In Paul's bedroom the cupboard door hung off its hinges because of being stuffed to bursting and slammed shut; his poor goldfish floated in its watery grave and his sports kit fermented in its wet and mouldy bag.

Louise's room had cake in the knicker drawer and pizza under the bed. Boy band posters hung on the walls and doors, and a nude but 'tasteful' Keanu Reeves was pasted on the inside of the wardrobe door.

In Clare's room the wallpaper lay in budgerigar chewed fragments on the floor, the guinea pig scuttled under the bed to put his little teeth through the bedside lamp wiring and the box in her room where we had attempted to grow mushrooms had been commandeered by the cat, as a litter tray.

Jane's bedroom, however, was as spotlessly clean and tidy as a showroom.

Every Wednesday Kate had a lady who helped her clean the house. Kate knew the phrase "Pam's coming today" would always get a mad scramble from Louise, Paul, and Clare to tidy up, while Jane hummed around her room flicking it over with a little duster.

Pam had been a WREN in the Royal Navy and loved everything to be Ship-Shape and Bristol Fashion. "Clear the decks" was a favourite saying of Pam's. Anything lying on the floor was automatically rubbish and was hoovered up every Wednesday.

Jane had a small appetite and asked for small portions at mealtimes, so Kate served literally, one pea, a postage stamp sized piece of meat and a teaspoon of potato. To the astonished gaze of guests, Kate would say: "She can always have second helpings." Home-made chocolate mousse, however, was in a different category. Jane took her own time eating and often slid under the dining table to either feed Charlotte the dog or put the remains from her plate into her pocket.

97

Jane took a very early aversion to public transport when, returning home from senior school on the double decker service bus, laden with hockey stick, boots and a large beef stew made in home economics, she fell from the top of the stairs and landed in a heap, much to the delight of the boys from the Grammar School. From then on Jane decided that public transport was to be avoided at all costs.

This came to light one day when Kate ordered a taxi to take herself and Jane to the railway station. "You found the house OK then?" Kate enquired of the driver.

"Oh, yes, *'course* I did," the taxi driver smiled, "Jane and I are *old* friends, aren't we!" Jane stared straight ahead.

Jane did well in school, went to university in Cardiff and there made friends with a group of girls with whom she has kept in touch to this day.

13. Kate Goes to India

IN 1976 WE got word that my younger brother Krishan was to get married. The custom is for both the bride's family and the groom's to invite everyone they know, and so the guest list can run into two or three hundred. This was an ideal opportunity for me to introduce Kate and our two children Louise and Paul, five and three years old respectively, to my family and friends.

The wedding was in November when the weather would be sunny but pleasantly cool. We took a flight from Heathrow to Frankfurt and then on to Delhi. We arrived at 4am, but nevertheless Kate had changed into a sari *en route* and looked bandbox fresh as she stepped onto Indian soil and into Palam Airport.

"This place is like my Dad's packing shed!" she exclaimed as she looked up at the roof rafters, then down at the concrete floor. Pigeons flew about among the ceiling fans. Kate ushered the children round sleeping passengers stretched out on the floor, as we made our way to the Customs Desk.

Airport officials in India wear military-style khaki uniforms. Kate remarked: "Only Indian women could make a khaki shirt and a pair of baggy trousers look elegant!" In the Arrivals Hall, my Father and two of my brothers were frantically waving from the first-floor gallery.

We emerged blinking onto the 6am Street. Delhi was already awake. A rickshaw stand was parked up like a taxi rank outside the airport, the cyclists stretched out like stiff planks with feet on the handlebars and head on the saddle; they were snoozing under a Government sign that said *Discipline: The Need of the Hour*. "We'll take a taxi to Le Meridian and order breakfast," my Father said. He whispered to me: "Dacoits put up road-blocks to catch taxis meeting these international flights." (Dacoits are bandits.) He added, "We can move on when the sun comes up." Under the glittering chandelier and beside the cascading waterfall, was where we took breakfast; India certainly is a land of contrasts. Dawn broke and we left for my hometown.

"This is like a sitting room," said Louise as she settled in the back seat of the taxi. Strings of tinsel, chillies and marigolds hung from the ceiling and around the doors of the taxi. At the windows were pink net curtains and a joss stick on the dashboard was alight with fragrant smoke. Also on the dashboard was a picture of Guru Nanak with his half-closed eyes and long white beard, his hand raised in blessing, and the Hindu God Shiva, his eight arms and legs pointing in different directions.

We drove steadily along the sprawling outskirts of Delhi, over the railway crossing and onto the Grand Trunk Road, which would take us forty miles north to Meerut. The road was busy with Ambassadors, India's own brand of car, and scooters crammed with four passengers, whilst brightly painted lorries spectacularly veered all over the road under the weight of their cargo. The lorries were painted with baskets of flowers, peacocks, climbing roses and watering cans, and tattered strings of tinsel, tied front and back, glittered in the sunshine. On the tailgate of each lorry was always painted: *Horn Please, OK. Tata.*

Kate was curious and I explained that Tata is a manufacturer of heavy plant, machinery and lorries and *Horn Please* is a request to alert the driver that you are about to overtake. A blast on the horn is not considered bad road manners in India. We left the outskirts of Delhi and traffic became less.

We now passed small fertile fields, growing green vegetables such as spinach and mustard. Sugar cane, eight

100

feet tall, cast shadows across the road. In the fields, buffalo pulled ploughs, churning the rich soil into furrows. We passed the occasional roadside café, set out with chairs and tables under jute tarpaulins.

Louise and Paul were now fast asleep, as we picked up speed and bounced along the wide, but potholed, road. The traffic further thinned to a few cars and motorbikes; occasionally the odd cyclist wobbled onto the road and then just as quickly disappeared again.

Long-distance lorries, some of them hurtling towards us down the wrong side of the road, were the only thing keeping our driver awake now. Ancient wooden buffalo carts, piled high with sugar cane, passed by on their way to the small village sugar refineries.

We had travelled about twenty-five miles when our driver suddenly stopped. "Puncture!" he said as he threw open his door. He stood at the side of the road, eating peanuts. Half-an-hour passed, then he hailed a taxi driver friend travelling in the opposite direction. His friend pulled his spare tyre from his boot and the two of them replaced our damaged one. The friend took the punctured tyre with him for repair. Such camaraderie was great to see, but the tyre we replaced was as bald as the tyre we took off.

We stopped again for a drink and light refreshment at The Ganga roadside cafe. Two more hours and we reached Meerut.

The Mehta family home is at the end of a quiet cul-de-sac. My Mother had been waiting for us since early morning. She stood in the middle of the road in the mid-morning sunshine, her shawl wrapped around her. Her face broke into a wide smile and her arms opened in greeting as soon as she saw us. The whole street hung over their garden gates, curious to see Kate, my English wife, and my children. I bent forward and touched my mother's feet and she patted me on my head and gave a blessing. Then Kate did the same and Mother gave her a big hug. It was an emotional moment, and we were overwhelmed to see the tears of joy on her cheeks.

As usual in India, everyone feels free to participate in anything going on, so I knew soon there would be a steady trickle of visitors. My Mother hugged Louise and Paul and ushered us into the house. My sister Shashi had died suddenly whilst I had been away, and I was very sad to be in the house without her there. It would have seemed the most natural thing in the world if she had walked over to hug me and meet Kate and our children for the first time.

Mother had made Indian chai with aniseed, green cardamom, cloves, stem ginger, water, tea leaves, milk and sugar all boiled up together and strained. We had tea with biscuits, almonds and chickoo, a fruit that is easily digested. As we had had a long journey, my Mother insisted we had a rest, and she would stand gatekeeper and keep visiting neighbours at bay.

We woke up early morning to the nasal cry of the vegetable seller in the street. I could see his handcart piled high with spinach and white radish, all draped with a piece of wet hessian sack to keep it moist in the dry heat of the sun. Mother had someone in to do the laundry and we could hear her slapping and beating the clothes on a flat stone in the wash-room downstairs. A knock on the door, and there stood Mother with a morning cup of tea. My younger brother brought a kettle full of boiling water to our upstairs washroom, which we mixed with the cold water in a bucket to wash.

Kate and the children were the talk of the neighbourhood and everybody wanted to meet them. We were guests of the whole road and invitations to visit factories, the dairy farm, the cinema, schools, and weddings came in abundance. The owner of Queens Bakery was very keen to show us his bakery and I was sure we would enjoy a visit there.

Kate gathered up Louise and Paul in one hand and her sari skirts in the other, and we went along. The shop was on one side of the street and the bakery was directly opposite. We entered directly from the street through a narrow doorway. It was dark inside; all we could see were the ovens with fires beneath. The flames glowed and we could feel the heat. The walls were covered in smoke-blackened grease. Three master bakers crouched on the floor, wearing tattered vests and cloths round their heads to act as a pad for carrying trays of cakes. They had no shoes. Their skin glistened in the firelight.

The trays went into the ovens on long-handled shovels and re-emerged ten minutes later, transformed into light, crisp, golden confectionery. The whole operation was performed with a dexterity and slickness borne of long practice in their specialised field. Dozens of trays full of golden bread buns, fresh out of the oven, were laid out on the earthen floor and feather-light sponge cakes, decorated with fresh cream, nestled in boxes on the table.

In the flickering light, we saw steps ascending one wall and disappearing through an opening in the ceiling. The steps were worn away in the middle and years of use had carved out little finger holds in the grimy wall, in the absence of any rail or banister. Halfway up the stairs a little landing with a door at the far end was where the flour was hauled up in jute sacks. Further upstairs was a room where the light streamed in a thin ribbon from a window at one end. There, in the middle, was a long table. Two bakers were busy icing birthday cakes in green and red. We came away with two large boxes of the best confectionery this side of Delhi.

It was the custom in our family that, after the evening meal, we would take a stroll down the street to the Paan stall. Paan is a mix of menthol, lime, betel nut, crushed mango, ginger, and cardamom, all wrapped in green Paan leaf. The Paan maker was in the same place, his hand cart parked in the market and lit by two hissing paraffin lamps suspended above. He was sitting cross-legged, bare feet in the Paan leaves, and his question was always the same: "Sweet or Tobacco?"

I had been friends with Kawal and Bina Loria all my life. Kawal and his father before him were skilled and highly regarded surgeons on Begum Bridge. Before I went to medical school, I enjoyed dropping into their surgery to talk to them, discussing medicine and the possibility of going abroad to do post-graduation. Kawal had been to America.

We were invited to their house. It was a spacious house with lilies, roses, and jasmine outside in the garden. Bina had trained as a nurse in South India. We had tea with them and were joined by Kawal's lovely hundred-and-one-year-old mother. She was a remarkable woman; she read several newspapers every day and knew what was happening around the world. We had a great discussion, and it was lovely to see them.

My brothers Krishan and Ravi arranged for Kate, myself, and the children to visit the Military Dairy Farm. We were welcomed by the manager who conducted us around his spotlessly clean Milking Parlour. The cows were lovingly cared for and in great health. "These ladies," the manager said with a wave of his arm towards his cows contentedly chewing hay, "we play classical music for them while they are being milked." He smiled. "Ah yes, they don't like pop, we tried it." He showed us how they made cheese and then he poured each one of us a glass of the freshest milk we are ever likely to have. The farm had a courtyard where the cows could gather under the shade of a large tree when brought in from the field. A flower garden surrounded the milking parlour and the entrance driveway. We thanked the manager for the wonderful visit and said goodbye to the contented cows.

My youngest brother Ravi made plans to show us a small flour mill. To see it working, we had to be there at the crack of dawn. We were welcomed by the owner, who showed Kate and me how the grinding of wheat and other cereals is done using a millstone. The mill and the millers were all in white, covered in flour dust but spotlessly clean.

We were invited to a small sugar factory on the outskirts of the town. The area around Meerut grows sugar cane in abundance. On the way there, we passed half a dozen heavy wooden bullock carts laden with sugar cane, lined up on the road outside the factory gates waiting for it to be weighed and unloaded. The cane is chopped up in a lethal looking machine, its blades whirring just millimetres from the hands that feed it. Sunk into the ground were six large circular pans of boiling syrup. Crouched over each pan was a man with a large ladle, stirring slowly. Some of the workers had no shoes. Six clouds of steam rose from the bubbling inferno, each cauldron of syrup was bubbling away at 99 Centigrade (210 Fahrenheit). Our two small children stood well back, and we gripped their hands firmly. We saw raw sugar put into moulds, left to set, and sent to the markets.

We made our way past the factory office, dimly lit by a 40-watt bulb, said our goodbyes, and left with a sigh of relief.

My family was very keen that Kate should see the Taj Mahal in Agra, one of the Seven Wonders of the World. We took the Taj Express train to Agra. The train has spacious compartments, complimentary mineral water, newspapers, and tea with biscuits.

At the Taj, Kate was shown, with the utmost politeness, where the British had gouged precious stones from the walls and stole them. We marvelled at the architecture, the craftsmanship and the love story. The fountains played and the fragrant roses bloomed in the surrounding gardens. We were told all about Mumtaz Mahal, in whose memory this monument came to be built by her husband Shah Jahan. It was built as a tomb for her, and as a monument to his undying love.

Next day we took an internal flight in a small plane from Delhi to Jaipur to see my elder brother. "Aaah! Where is Daddy taking us now?" groaned Louise as she looked out of the airplane window and saw a vast expanse of red desert beneath. The Maharaja of Jaipur, very distinguished in his cream cashmere suit, sat next to us and had a pleasant conversation with Louise.

Jaipur in 1976 had a small airport with only three walls. The missing side was open onto the red sandy desert. We were collected by my brother. "This house is *your* house," he said, "We want you to feel at home." We went up on the flat roof and looked out over the magnificent wide expanse of desert, glowing red in the setting sun. "Ah, I must show you this," he said, pointing to a large, covered water tank. "This is filled once a day and when it's gone, it's gone. Clean your teeth in a mug of water and put a plug in the sink please, don't run the water."

In the morning, we went to the Fort, home to Maharajas in the past. The Fort housed the largest water urn in the world, made from silver. There were armaments, furniture and even the carpets used two centuries ago, all in pristine condition due to the almost zero humidity. We travelled in a rickshaw to see the Hawa Palace (Wind Palace)

106

"See?" said my brother Raj, "They had air conditioning here in the 18th century." He told us the palace was "built for the harem in 1799."

The Jaigarh Fort was high up on a hill overlooking Jaipur, and it took us half an hour to get there. The walls are thick, it was built to withstand an attack; from the tiny windows we looked out onto Maota Lake below, glistening in the noonday heat. The lake was the fort's water supply. On a visit here a few years later, Clare, then aged three, sat in her pushchair and was about to eat an orange when an elephant behind her reached over her shoulder, robbed her of her orange and popped it in its own mouth. Far from being amused, Clare scolded it!

Rajasthani men are recognisable by their big moustaches, large turbans and pointed shoes. The women wear long skirts, often with tiny mirrors embroidered on, a tight bodice and a cloth over the head, with one end tucked into the waistband. It is tradition for Rajasthani women to wear heavy jewellery. Women wear rings and pendants on toes, ankles, fingers, arms, nose, ears, and forehead. Men wear rings in ears and on fingers.

We returned home for the wedding. An Indian wedding lasts for four or five days and the ladies dress in an array of beautiful saris. Kate had brought a sari from England: it was blue and embroidered with silver. The women of our family dressed and got themselves ready in our dark and tiny bedroom. With one fifteen-centimetre mirror hanging on the wall, it was a case of everyone helping everyone else.

Kate's sari did not meet with approval. "Wrong colour," they said. So a red and gold sari was generously loaned and fitted on. "Wrong jewellery now." And some real gold bling was fastened round her neck, ears, wrists, and head. Kate was having fun as the sisters-in-law got to

107

transforming her. "Make-up's too light," they said, as they rolled up their sleeves and Kate lay back on the bed, closed her eyes and submitted to the complete works. The sisters stood back to admire their handiwork as Kate emerged into the sunshine, a glittering Bollywood lookalike.

"Well," she whispered, "what do you think?" I could not believe my eyes, somewhere under there was my Kate!

"OK for here," I said, "and *they're* happy," I nodded towards the approving sisters-in- law, "but not in Wakefield."

My brother Krishan, the Groom, went to fetch his bride on a white horse. He rode up to her door in his new suit and a traditional turban strewn about with marigold flower-heads. A band played in the street and all 150 of us danced our way behind Krishan and the horse, to the bride's house and the ceremony. On reaching the bride's house, we were greeted by her family, so there were three hundred of us now, the men hugging and back- slapping, the ladies being rather more genteel. We were escorted to the marquee and the band played on. We were invited for a drink and settled down for the wedding ceremony.

Kate, the children and I had seats at the front so I could explain the proceedings. A sacred fire was lit in a little brazier. The bride and groom are tied to each other with a sacred scarf and walk round the fire four times. The bride was very beautiful and very shy, as befits an Indian bride. She was dressed in a magenta-coloured sari embroidered with gold. She walked slowly and gracefully and kept her eyes downcast all day. Her name Sneh, which means Love, from this day forth would be loved by Krishan and our family for ever more.

We visited India every two or three years to see my parents. As the children grew up and left home, Kate and I visited India on our own.

Mother was still active in the community, both politically and in her charity work. She decided that, during our stay, I should give something back to the country that trained me. An MBBS (Bachelor of Medicine, Bachelor of Surgery) is the most expensive university degree anywhere in the world. I also have a degree in Zoology. I won scholarships for all my schooling and both my universities. My parents were proud of all their children's academic achievements despite the great adversity we suffered.

My Mother usually phoned the local Community Centre and volunteered my services. I always travel to India equipped with medical supplies as I know they will be needed. The Pundit at the Community Centre asked, "Can you come tomorrow at six?" "Yes, that's fine," I replied, "Great! An early start then, we'll have about a hundred for you to see!" He explained: "We've let everyone in the community know, the school and the orphanage too."

So Kate and I started early the next day. I checked everyone; and those we found needing medical help, I either gave the treatment straight away, or a note to see their regular doctor. Kate was kept busy writing notes, washing instruments, and giving out an orange to each little patient. Sadly, some were very seriously ill, brought in on stretchers, but we saw them all.

A travel agent friend organised a short trip for us to Khajuraho in Madhya Pradesh (Middle Province). It was a special deal he had going. The main attraction is a group of five temples, built in the ninth century and carved from top to bottom with erotic carvings.

The Chandalas, a religious sect, lived there and put up these edifices depicting sacred carnal activity of every kind. It certainly was a labour of love, considering it was all done with a hammer and chisel whilst balancing on bamboo

109

scaffolding. The Chandalas believed that sexual activity was a form of worship. The carvings included Vishnu enfolded in the coils of the eternal serpent and Lord Krishna dancing with his devotees: nine young, unmarried cow-herd girls known as Gopis. Human forms entwined in every way imaginable were also carved into the outer stone walls of the temples.

Our favourite hotel is The Imperial near Connaught Place in Delhi. This is where some political meetings were held in the 1940s as part of the *Quit India* campaign culminating in India's Independence in 1947. Mahatma Gandhi attended the meetings but refused to stay in such luxurious surroundings. He slept in a sweeper's hut nearby. Built in 1936, The Imperial was designed to be one of the finest monuments of Lutyens's grand vision of the capital city's building plan, presenting a blend of Victorian, Old Colonial and Art Deco styles. The building encloses a garden with scented roses and jasmine and a shady lawn set with small tables and wicker chairs, where turbaned waiters bring afternoon tea. The place was gently crumbling away; we loved its high ceilings, its ancient plumbing, and its gracious staff.

Our room was spacious; the shutters on the long windows shaded the midday sun, the ceiling fan whirred above the enormous bed and the bathroom was reassuringly old fashioned. Kate decided on a bath before dinner; but as quickly as the water ran into the old roll-top bath, it ran out along the concrete floor towards the drain.

We decided not to call for maintenance, as we imagined the man arriving with a bucket and trowel and plying the hole with wet cement for at least a day. We plugged the hole with the bath towel and increased the flow from the beautiful brass taps and managed well for the next three days. The Imperial has now been renovated and become a modern five-star hotel; but in so doing, has lost its faded charm from a bygone age.

I sometimes felt I was also of a bygone age. My hair was turning grey and becoming much thinner. At that time there appeared in the newspaper an advertisement for a revolutionary new remedy for hair loss, and bottles of it were apparently 'flying off the shelf.' The advertisement told of redundant hair follicles brought back to life. One of my bald friends tried the treatment and found some success so he recommended a hairdresser in the town who was selling it.

I had arranged to visit my family in India and the previous time they saw me, I had a mop of black hair, so Kate decided that I should have a bottle of this treatment and also get my hair dyed. She made an appointment. A quick consultation with a medical practitioner at the salon told me I was a suitable candidate. He handed me a brown glass bottle of the solution to rub into my scalp twice a day.

Back at home I poured a little of the magic potion into my cupped hands and waited for the promised hair to appear. "Crikey Dad," grinned Paul as he peered round the bathroom door one morning, "you've got more on your hands than your head" he added "you'll still have a bald head, but lovely hairy hands!"

Then Kate booked an appointment with the hairdresser. She explained that I needed a total hair makeover. "We'll do our best," they said, "We'd better book him with the boss." So I had my hair dyed jet black, then at the end of the treatment he fluffed my hair so much that my head looked like a giant black crow's nest.

I had to go straight back to the hospital from there, so my son collected me in the car. "Dad!" laughed Paul, "that's a great look! Hang on, I'll open the sunroof so we can get you in." He helpfully put a hand on my blown-up hair to squash it down so I could get in the car.

111

I saw several patients that afternoon who swore they had seen a more elderly surgeon the week before. Later that afternoon, as I was walking down the corridor, there was giggling behind me; one of my colleagues could not stop laughing. When I went to the consultants' sitting room first there was a studied silence; my colleagues tried to talk to me without grinning, their eyes straying ever upwards to my towering coiffure. My good friend broke the ice: "For God's sake Sat, what happened to you?" They all burst out laughing as my friend said: "You need urgent treatment for that! Can't think which department it might come under."

14. White Rose County

I STARTED MY job in Barnsley in 1977 on the same day that Barnsley and District General Hospital opened. The Beckett hospital, built in 1864 with only 154 beds, and St Helen's maternity hospital, built in 1930, were left vacant, a testament to the past, as staff re-located to the brand-new place about a mile away.

Everything in the new hospital, with a capacity of 850 beds, was the latest and most modern and there were new staff members too, including me. But it seemed it had escaped the notice of the committee responsible that, with more beds, we would need more equipment; and we struggled for months with a lack of both very basic and more specialised machines and medical instruments. There was a shortage of theatre instruments, so we were obliged to reduce our theatre lists and keep patients waiting for longer.

For those who don't know, Barnsley is between Sheffield and Leeds in the heart of the Yorkshire coal fields and many of my patients were pitmen or their families. I loved the warm and friendly ways, the generosity, and the family-orientated ethos that I found among the townspeople I had chosen to serve. I took to it immediately and Barnsley took to me. I liked the hint of old English in the dialect, as *thees* and *thous* peppered my patients' sentences.

From the outset, I ran my department on democratic lines. I was accessible to both patients and staff; my secretaries knew where I would be at any given time and my patients had my secretaries' contact numbers. As time went on, I acquired seven part-time secretaries. "Mrs Mehta," they said to Kate whenever they saw her, "Can't you take Mr Mehta away on a long holiday, just so we can catch up with some paperwork?" Seriously ill patients could admit themselves to my ward by ringing my secretary or Outpatient Sister. They could bring themselves in either day or night and knew they would find care and relief there.

We were a team and we worked as such. I gave lunchtime talks to the nursing staff, junior doctors, audio technicians and staff in the hearing-aid department. My talks were about ENT diseases and how to treat them. I talked about what happens in the operating theatre, and what the many laboratory results mean. The staff were happy to forego their lunch hour. They knew they had become vital in the running of the department; and the more they knew, the more our patients would benefit.

I had the privilege of having a team in the outpatient department, ward and theatre, who worked as a family, delivering the best care for our patients. There were no demarcation lines. I set up a Combined Clinic with a Consultant Oncologist (Cancer Specialist) from Sheffield and together with my ENT colleague, also a Consultant Histo-pathologist (laboratory tests) and a Consultant Maxilla-facial surgeon (Head and Neck surgeon) we made it possible for our patients with Cancer to have a consultation, be referred to any one of us, and have any tests or investigations done, all in the one visit.

Like anywhere else, patients addicted to drugs turned up in the clinic. Snorting Cocaine eventually causes the nasal septum to erode and a hole between the two nasal passages is the usual complaint, needing surgical repair. But a septal hole can also be the result of an injury such as a broken nose, so to suggest to a patient that snorting drugs has eroded their nasal septum can cause distress.

Addicted patients invariably do not mention their addiction until lying on the trolley in the anaesthetic room. Me and my team, scrubbed, masked and gowned, in the operating theatre ready to see the anaesthetised patient

114

wheeled in, would be halted by a nurse, who ran in from the anaesthetic room. "Mr Mehta!" The nurse would say, "Patient wants a word! Says it's urgent!" We both knew the reason as the nurse rolled her eyes. So, I would be called from the operating theatre and our tight schedule disrupted. In the anaesthetic room, the anaesthetist and I would hear the drug-related history. "I'm on coke, Doc."

"How much, how many lines a day?" I would ask.

"I dunno, two maybe three."

Frank, the anaesthetist, would say: "Where do you get it from, is it mixed with anything?" Before selling on the street, Cocaine can be mixed with flour, corn starch, or talcum powder to increase profits. On the other hand, and far more dangerous, it can be mixed with synthetic opioids, or a stimulant, to make the hallucinogenic effects more intense and faster acting.

"I dunno. I get it off Nuzzy. It works, it's good shit, that's all I know," would be a typical reply.

There is no way either the anaesthetist or I can know the quantity or quality of drug the patient takes. We only have their word and hazy recollections to go on. Frank and I would weigh up the risks and either cancel the operation or write up a much higher dose of morphine for after the op, to numb the pain. Higher doses of pain relief are needed as these patients have made themselves immune to lower, safer doses. These are the extra responsibilities we shoulder. If it all goes well, that is fine; if not, we are in court.

The few cases of HIV we suspected caused much confused medical protocol in those early days of the disease. No test for HIV was permitted without the patient's request. Furthermore, disclosure of HIV status to medical staff was entirely at the patient's discretion. This was obviously risky to hospital staff as we encountered patients' blood daily. I gave instructions that, if HIV were suspected, then staff

115

should wear two pairs of surgical gloves, one on top of the other. Needlestick injuries to hands was the most common cause for concern, and two pairs of gloves does not protect in that circumstance, so my directive was a forlorn hope.

HIV on the wards brought its problems too. One day a patient's husband crashed through the doors and thundered onto the ENT ward. His stocky frame, shaven head, massive, tattooed arms and neck gave him a menacing appearance. Rummaging around in drawers and cupboards at home, he had come across evidence of his wife's infidelity with their neighbour. It was rumoured the neighbour was HIV positive.

"Where's the stinkin' bitch? I'll kill her!" he roared at a passing nurse. His face was purple, and his fists clenched as he strode towards his wife's bed. Her diminutive frame cowered under the bedclothes.

He stopped short suddenly and uttered a thunderous "Aaaah!" He ripped the oxygen supply from the wall and threw it with a crash to the floor. Plaster fell in great lumps and splintered in pieces. Screws, bolts and tubing scattered across the polished floor. He then rounded angrily on his wife and put his hands round her neck

"You slut! Give *me* AIDS, would you?" he bellowed, "As well as you and your fancy man!" His wife coughed and spluttered as he battered her head repeatedly against the metal railing at the head of the bed. It took all six staff to drag him off the bed and land him on the floor. He got up and shook them off like flies.

Eventually, the calm, reasoned and authoritative voice of Ward Sister persuaded both wife and husband to take a blood test, which she instantly arranged. Luckily both tests proved negative; and, as far as I know, all ended well.

I was serving in Barnsley during the miners' strike of 1984-85. The National Union of Mineworkers HQ was in Barnsley and, during that time, it was busier than usual. Head of the Union was Arthur Scargill, born into a mining family in Worsborough Dale nearby. His father Harold had been a miner and member of the Communist Party of Great Britain.

The Union building is on a leafy street near the city centre, just north of the town hall. The stone building was known locally as King Arthur's Castle, on account of its ornate turrets, bay windows and double front door. Outside on the grass stands, a bronze statue of a miner in his helmet, knee pads and boots; beside him his barefoot wife cradling a baby, and on the other side a little girl. On the plinth is the inscription: 'IN MEMORY OF THOSE WHO HAVE LOST THEIR LIVES IN SUPPORTING THEIR UNION IN TIMES OF STRUGGLE.'

Owing to the strike, the hospital's main activity stopped for nine months. In support of the miners' strike, many hospital porters, electricians, staff sterilizing instruments and cleaning staff withdrew their services, leaving a skeleton staff to carry on. The accident and emergency department, hospital clinics, surgical and medical emergencies could be attended to, but routine cases could not be treated, and the waiting list shot up. All in all, a difficult time for everybody.

15. Friends

IN THE SUMMER of 1978, we moved into a family sized house with an acre of garden, on the outskirts of Wakefield, West Yorkshire. We began introducing ourselves to the neighbours. "Hello, I'm Sat Mehta we've just moved in, I'm your new neighbour" I called over the garden fence.

The next-door neighbour was mowing his lawn, but he gave no sign of having seen or heard me. I tried for ten minutes without success. The following day we introduced ourselves to the other side and mentioned that communication on the one side had been impossible. Our friendly neighbour said: "Aaah yes, he's deaf. He was a prisoner of war in Burma on the railway, you know. It's a wonder he survived at all. Japanese knocked him deaf with explosives and guns."

The next day Kate and I went across to his house and introduced ourselves. He told us he owned a factory producing hot water bottles, babies' dummies and the like. He never married and lived alone. One sad day Kate heard plaintive cries from behind his front door. Kate and another neighbour picked the lock and discovered him in a heap at the bottom of the stairs: he had suffered a stroke. He had been there for two days. He was taken to hospital and died a few days later.

In the house at the bottom of the garden lived Doug and Hilary. Doug was of Dutch descent but born and brought up in Tanzania, in Africa. He had worked for the Government Water Department, finding supplies of water and establishing tube wells for rural villages. They had now retired to Hilary's native Yorkshire. Doug's job took him and his team camping on the plains of Africa for weeks. He was used to an outdoor life, nothing to fence him in, going where the water courses took him, under the African sky. His retirement to Yorkshire meant his roaming days were over, but on any given evening Doug could be found sitting beside a small bonfire in his garden, gazing into the flames and re-living his days on the wide-open veld. Our gardens adjoined and so did our neighbour's on the other side, so we made two gates between us all, so Doug could keep us all safe with his evening patrols across our gardens and come and go as he pleased.

Whenever I had a bonfire in the orchard, I'd hear the gate click. "I've got some nice applewood for that, Sat," and Doug would sit down beside me, his beer in hand and chat until the embers died and it was well after dark. We loved to listen, sitting round the bonfire, to his stories of safari in deepest, wildest Africa, of how he saved a village from a lion who settled on the rooftops and refused to move, of snakes in the kitchen and termites in the hall.

Doug sent Hilary to live in the house a full five years before he arrived. The reason was, in Doug's own words: "You're too much of a liability, woman, I told you to shoot *at* him, not shoot him!" Doug chuckled as he remembered. "I was going away on a long trip, and I said to Hilary: *You keep this rifle by the door. If any of these young Morani (Kenyan warriors) get too friendly, point this at him, you know how to use it!*"

Doug had been gone a week or so when a young warrior did enter Hilary's kitchen and, in spite of Hilary's "Don't come any nearer, or I'll shoot, I will!" he advanced forward, so Hilary shot him in the leg.

He hopped away and returned with his friend who asked to borrow Hilary's Jeep to take the young man to hospital. "Certainly not!" said Hilary "I'll never see it again! Come over here and I'll dig the bullet out" And that is exactly what happened.

Hilary was reported to the police in Nairobi and had to appear in court. "What happened then, Doug?" thrilled as we were to hear the story, Doug growled and said "Nothing, she was bound over to keep the peace for six months, but I thought she and the boys are better off out of it, so I sent them to England." So, we made a mental note *never* to upset Hilary.

Doug was very protective to everyone around him. He was in his bedroom one night when he heard breaking glass and saw a burglar breaking and entering into the young couple next-door. The occupants were petrified and cowered behind the curtains, but Doug grabbed his five-foot-long spear off the wall and, with a mighty battle cry, charged through his neighbour's front door and the burglar fled for his life.

I had never been fishing till I met Doug. I was given fishing tackle on my retirement from the hospital and had learnt how to cast a line. Four of us decided to go to County Mayo in Ireland to catch salmon. We fished near a bridge, made famous because Jackie Charlton had once fished there. We discussed our fishing successes and failures every night in the pub; everyone else in the pub was doing the same. We celebrated our successes in pints of Guinness and went to bed on a tot of Irish whiskey.

"There's a drumming festival in Angus, in the highlands of Scotland," said Kate "I'd like to go. Fancy coming along?' The drumming festivals that Kate goes to tend be held in remote places. African drumming is not to everyone's taste, including mine, so I said: "Yes, I'll come with you, but you go drumming and I'll go fishing." I found a remote loch where silver birch branches hung low and dipped into the water's edge. Fish jumped up to catch gnats dancing on the water's surface and kingfishers sat on branches and studied the waters beneath. I knew I had found a great spot. I arranged my fishing gear, rods and net for a few hours quiet fishing. I could see some birds circling in the sky.

As soon I cast my line, I heard the whoosh of wings above my head. I looked up to see a score or more birds of prey circling my head. My second casting caused a real stir: I was dive bombed from above, as the birds skimmed my head. I ducked when one, bolder than the rest, gave me a glancing scratch with his talons, on my bald head. I was alone on the lock and these birds were not going to let me take their fish. I am not good at recognising birds but after discussing with Kate and a few other people, we concluded these were Ospreys.

Andy is a good family friend. His family has a farm and Andy manages the farm, repairs farm machinery, builds barns and generally deals with all things agricultural. He skilfully converted some old stone barns into cottages and lived in the large cottage himself.

He preserved the beamed ceilings and stone flagged floor. He installed pipes underneath the floor to carry the central heating, had a proper subterranean pantry with a large cold slab, and he preserved many of the original nooks and crannies from a bygone era. We are very fond of him and he joins us sometimes on bonfire nights and other functions. We seek his advice regarding trees, fridges, cars and good food.

Andy had a share in a four-seater fixed wing aeroplane. His partner was not in good health and no longer flew, so Andy had exclusive use of the aeroplane.

Kate and I have always been enthralled by aviation and when Andy offered us a flight, we jumped at it. "It's easy!" he explained as Kate strapped herself into the

121

front passenger seat. Andy pushed the joystick "go up, go down, go left, go right!"

I got behind with my video camera. "Open the window, Sat!" advised Andy, "You'll get a better view for the camera." We flew from one small airfield to another, we flew round Lincolnshire, Nottinghamshire and most of Yorkshire. Andy called up on the crackling radio to arrange our next stop. It was thrilling to touch down on the runways and go into the Portacabins to have a mug of tea and talk with the pilots. We examined maps, filled in logbooks and checked the weather.

We flew over Doncaster, saw Ferry Bridge Cooling Towers, followed the River Humber, glistening in the sunshine all the way to the east coast. We took a turn inland and rang our children to put white sheets on the lawn, in the shape of an X. We flew over our house and the children jumped up and down, waving enthusiastically as we repeatedly circled the rooftops. We dipped and looped, it was exhilarating, a thrilling adventure, and then we began to feel sick!

Andy, however, was just getting started. He assured us the plane could do acrobatics and we swung west to circle Walton Hall and its beautiful lake. I leaned out the window and recorded our dips and loops to show the children when we got home. We took a deep dive over Andy's parent's house and then headed back to the airfield.

We had spent the whole day up in the wide blue yonder, defying gravity and marvelling at the beauty below. It was a truly amazing day. A treat like that would have cost a fortune, if we had taken a Red Letter Experience Day.

We came home and watched the whole thing all over again on the TV, had a meal and went to bed. It was, without a doubt, one of the best days of excitement we have ever experienced.

16. Tales from Barnsley

MY HOSPITAL LIFE in Barnsley proved exceptionally hectic and varied. Here are a few of the cases I remember best.

One Christmas Day, an eighty-year-old man *walked* into the A&E Department with a bread knife through his neck. He had run it in with such force that it entered in the front, and the tip was buried somewhere in the back of his neck. He had obviously attempted suicide. The casualty officer was understandably concerned and immediately rang me.

I needed to find the path the blade had taken and see if any vital structures had been damaged. I could see the knife had entered near the trachea that carries air from the larynx to the lungs and followed a straight line through to the spinal vertebrae at the back.

I asked for six pints of blood to be grouped and cross-matched, so that the donor's blood would be compatible with my patient's blood and put on standby in the Blood Bank. I then arranged the emergency theatre and an anaesthetist. I would have to remove the blade under X-Ray control, so I had to call the Radiographer out too.

On the operating table, I used the suction machine to clear the blood away. The X-Ray showed the tip of the blade had pierced a vertebrae bone and had become embedded there. I very carefully followed the track the knife took, enlarging the entry wound and sealing off the bleeding points with an electric current. I found the blade had just missed the larynx, the trachea, the carotid artery supplying the brain with blood, and the nerves of the upper spinal cord running along the inside of the vertebrae. When I reached the vertebrae, I moved the knife vertically, gently dislodging

123

the tip. I finally withdrew the knife from the wound, checked the area again, inserted a vacuum drain and closed the wound in layers.

In the Recovery Room, I checked the patient's legs for any sign of neurological damage that might have been caused by injury to his spinal cord. I kept the patient in the Intensive Care Unit for 24 hours, then transferred him to my ward for a few days. We looked after him with gentleness and, on discharge, we arranged for social service help with his loneliness.

When he came for his follow-up clinic appointment, he brought a box of chocolates. "I'm really sorry about what I did," he said, "I was depressed, and Christmas Day just got on top of me. My family are fighting between themselves and life just seemed a mess."

I said: "I hope things have improved since I last saw you. The wound has healed well and there is no lasting damage to your neck."

Another Christmas story. The parents of a 13-year-old boy gave him an airgun for Christmas. The boy was delighted, and his younger brother could not wait to join in the fun too.

The day after Boxing Day, the boys were left alone in the house whilst the parents went to visit some friends. The boys opened the airgun box. On the lounge floor, they arranged three thick Telephone Directories. They then balanced the airgun on the top. The younger one was directed to lie on the floor, whilst his brother lined him up along the barrel of the gun. They then placed an apple in his mouth, clenched between his front teeth, as a target. The elder brother pulled the trigger. *Crack!* The airgun hit the apple. But the boys did not realise the airgun would be so powerful. They thought the pellet would become embedded in the apple. The pellet in fact went straight through the

124

apple and into the back of the younger brother's throat. The younger one screamed with surprise and pain. His throat bled profusely, and he started showing signs of shock.

The elder brother phoned his parents. They arrived home to find their eldest son distraught and their younger son spurting blood from his mouth into a pool on the sitting room carpet. The boy was making gurgling sounds as the blood was pumping out faster than he could swallow it. The parents rushed with the little boy to our A&E department where I was waiting, together with my junior doctor. We arranged X-Rays of the neck and sent his blood for group and cross matching in the Blood Bank. His parents then signed a consent form for an emergency operation and we took him to the theatre.

The neck is a confined area funnelling vital nerves and blood vessels from the heart to and from the brain and the rest of the body. It is the "Clapham Junction" of the body and injury to this area results in very serious consequences. I asked for complete silence in the theatre. We called the radiographer again, this time to bring the mobile X-Ray machine into the theatre, as the pellet was not at the back of the throat.

We took more X-Rays from every angle we could. At last, the pellet was clearly visible. It had hit the spine, a cervical vertebra at the back of the neck. The pellet had then ricocheted and shot off to lodge near the carotid artery supplying the brain. I explored the neck with meticulous care. Under X-Ray control and using the magnifying microscope, I carefully lifted the pellet from beside the pulsating carotid where it had embedded in the tissues. We all sighed with relief as I dropped the pellet into a metal bowl!

I inserted a drain and closed the neck with stitches. Amazingly, the boy had sustained no permanent damage to any vital structures. I sent him to Intensive Care and went to tell his parents the happy news. The boy recovered completely.

Early one morning, as I was scrubbing up in the hospital operating theatre to start my list, a nurse came running in. "Where's Mr Mehta?" she shouted, "We need him in A&E. Now!"

Theatre Sister came to find me. The nurse added: "We've got a guy choking to death!" as I flung open the theatre doors and hurried down the corridor. I rounded the corner into A&E and made straight for the commotion behind the curtains at the far end of the department, my green operating gown flapping behind me.

The throng around him parted and I saw a man, his face purple and his eyes streaming, clutching his throat, his tongue out, choking and gasping for breath. He was desperately pushing away all the staff.

"He was eating a sandwich," his wife told me, "when suddenly he started to retch. He was mixing a chemical into his compost and some must have got onto his sandwich." She added: "We've come straight from the allotment and this is..." She was about to hand me the bag of chemical, but I said: "We'll take him to theatre right now and help him to breathe." I added, as we wheeled him away: "You just hold on to that bag of chemical – we'll look at it later."

Sister took the wife's hand and said: "Doctor has got to go, love. He'll see you later when your husband's on the ward."

It took the anaesthetist, a nurse, and a porter to forcibly hold the oxygen mask on the patient's face as we ran him to the operating theatre on the trolley. We could not get into my theatre because my junior doctor had started my list of cases in my absence. Our choking patient was losing

126

consciousness and had turned blue. We wheeled him into the anaesthetic room. I felt for the rings of his trachea, stuck my knife in and twisted it round. The fastest tracheostomy possible! No gloves, gown, anaesthetic, or skin preparation! But the patient drew in a huge whistling breath and the colour began to return to his face. Saved in the nick of time, he sank back onto the blood-stained pillow.

I sealed off the bleeding points and inserted the tracheostomy tube. We injected him with painkillers and antibiotics and sent him back to the ward. The laboratory ran a sample of the chemical. He had suffered a severe reaction to it, but it had not burnt his oesophagus or trachea. I removed the tracheostomy tube and closed the hole after 48 hours. He could breathe easily, and his voice returned to normal, so I discharged him home.

A very unusual case walked into the A&E Department one day. The man was in great distress. At the desk, he could not tell the nurse what was wrong, but he pointed in agitation to his throat. He dribbled and retched, and so I was called.

On examination I saw that his whole upper denture was firmly wedged in his throat and was too big to remove easily. I arranged the case with theatre, and I got an anaesthetist. Once the patient was asleep, I propped his mouth open as widely as possible and tried to wriggle the denture free, but the surrounding tissues had become irritated and swollen. I packed behind the denture with wet gauze, then I called for a small electric saw. I cut the denture into small pieces and removed it in bits. I sent him back to the ward and discharged him the following day.

A little girl of four, who had difficulty in breathing and swallowing, was admitted to the children's ward. She was there for two days, being treated for either asthma or a severe throat infection. When she failed to respond to the treatment, I was called.

I sent her for an X-Ray and there, lodged deep in her throat, was a wooden clothes-peg with a metal spring. The peg lay so that one wooden prong stretched down her larynx and the other stretched down her oesophagus. I transferred her to my ward and took her to the operating theatre.

Clearly, she would be better once the peg was removed. In the operating theatre I removed the peg with great care, as the surrounding tissues had become swollen and inflamed. I lifted the peg carefully, first from the food pipe and then from the windpipe. I put her in the Intensive Care Ward for two days and she made a complete recovery.

One of my friends at the hospital was the Paediatrician, a specialist in children's diseases. He asked me to see a child whom he suspected of being physically and mentally abused. The boy came to my clinic accompanied by his mother. He was a small seven-year-old, very distressed and nervous, backing away from letting me look in his ears. According to his mother, he suffered severe pain in both ears.

We talked for a while and I said: "Don't worry. I'll stop if the examination hurts you." Very gently, I shone the auroscope in his ears and I found a large, ragged hole in his right ear drum. With the severity of the pain and the absence of any previous ear infections, there was no doubt this was the result of a sharp instrument pushed forcibly into the ears. The eardrum had a large perforation that was too big for me to mend. I found this case very distressing.

I was called to give my findings in court. My professional opinion of the injury and the reasons that led me to that opinion were considered by the judge. The trial revealed the child's mother had consistently injured her little boy over the years; and on this occasion, she admitted she had used a knitting needle. The little boy was taken into council care and his mother was sent for a psychiatric assessment.

In hospitals years ago, patients did not go home after treatment as quickly as they do nowadays, so Christmas had to be as special as we could make it. Furthermore, more than half of the young junior doctors were from overseas and lived on the hospital grounds in the Doctor's Residences. The majority of nurses also lived within the hospital grounds, in the Nurses' Homes.

The senior Nursing Sisters were often single and 'married' to their profession and the Consultants were at hospital more often than at home. The hospital in festive mode was, therefore, a place of comfort and joy for the senior staff and patients and an excuse for high jinks for the junior staff and students.

A small room in each ward and department was set aside for staff festivities. Ward and departmental Nursing Sisters organised food and drink and made sure of a good time, within sensible limits. In my junior doctor days, we were very careful to make sure on-duty staff stayed tee-total whilst the rest of us roamed the hospital, 'visiting.'

We visiting *roamers* sought out the 'party rooms' and were welcomed in with weak fruit punch, sausage rolls and mince pies. We ate and drank our way round the hospital, spreading our cheer and goodwill to all. Later, it would be our turn to stay sober to look after the patients.

When I became the ENT Department's Senior Consultant Surgeon, I was on the ward to carve the turkey on Christmas Day. I'd be accompanied by Kate and the children. As I had a children's ward as well as an adult ward, I had fun appearing on the wards as a pink and yellow spotted Mr. Blobby, a bright green Kermit the Frog or a one-eyed Pudsey Bear. We really tried to get the children home for Christmas, but there were usually four or five who had to stay with us.

The Operating Theatre Staff are kept busy over Christmas with emergencies. Operating lists run until December 23rd and resume again on about the 28th December. In a small reception room, the Staff had put together a wonderful scene from the fairy tale Cinderella. A large shop mannequin was brought in to be Cinderella, dressed in a blue and silver gown. She sat in her golden pumpkin-shaped coach and a life-size horse, complete with eyes, ears and a big swishy tail was harnessed to the coach. The carriage and horse were made from Plaster of Paris. The carriage was covered in Christmas lights and gold and silver threads. It looked fantastic and everyone enjoyed it, particularly the children.

I thought it was too good to dismantle after Christmas and the theatre staff offered it to me. The coach was too big to take, but I could take the horse home for my own four children and our friends and neighbour's children to enjoy.

Amused patients watched as theatre staff and I carried the horse through the hospital reception and into the car park, to the back of my estate car. "Wind the window down, Mr Mehta, his legs are going to have to stick out" advised the porter. The head of the horse rested on the dashboard, staring out through the windscreen; his front legs stuck out the front passenger side window, whilst his back legs dangled from the tailgate.

I headed for home, but I stopped at a newsagent shop, parking the car in a lay-by. On my returning to the car, a police car had stopped behind me and the constables were waiting. When they saw me coming, they got out of the police car and strode over. "Good afternoon Sir, is this your vehicle?"

"Yes" I replied.

"Have you got a horse in there?"

"Yes" I replied again.

They hurried over to my car and peered inside. "How did you acquire this horse, sir?"

I explained the hospital dismantled their Christmas decorations and the horse was going to my home for the children. "We're glad you're not carting around a dead horse, sir, had to check it out." They added: "Thank you. You're free to go!"

As they turned to go, I caught their walkie-talkie conversation with the Police Station, "No Sarge, it's *not* Shergar, *looked* like Shergar, this one's made of plaster." They added, "Yes Sarge, we've let the driver go."

(For those of my readers too young to know, Shergar was an Irish racehorse. He won every race he entered and was worth millions of pounds. He disappeared in mysterious circumstances and was never found.)

I continued my journey home with no more ado. The horse was received by the children with whoops of joy and admiration.

There were always more children at our house than our own four. Neighbours' children and friends' children would be either staying the night, come over for supper and to watch TV, or just passing through. In the summer we even put tents in the garden.

Anyway, "Shergar" had many admirers, and they decided that anyone over four years old was too big to ride him. Clare and Jane were declared the jockeys and hoisted unceremoniously onto his back. Shergar lived in the dining-room until eventually he crumbled away.

17. Unusual Cases

SUMMER IN ENGLAND is a wonderful vista of green trees, wildflowers and hedgerows. Fields bask in the sun and occasionally summer showers refresh the valleys, streets and parks with gentle rain.

But this profusion of nature's bounty comes at a price for some people. The air is filled with pollen from grasses, trees and flowers. My nose itched, my eyes watered, and I began to sneeze: I had developed hay fever.

I was working in ENT and took an interest in allergies. Genetically modified plants produce much stronger pollen-causing allergies. Sensitisation to pollen takes about seven to ten years to develop. Yorkshire had a history of coalmines, steelmaking, textiles and agriculture and these activities added further pollutants to the atmosphere and caused more complicated allergies. Nasal polyps are a result of chronic allergies. Polyps are growths that look like a bunch of grapes. I saw a number of these cases with polyps big enough to cause an obstruction of the nasal passages. In these circumstances the patient has no alternative but to breathe through the mouth. On examination, I would see not only the nose blocked but also a mass of polyps hanging down into the back of the throat. The polyps need to be gently removed under anaesthesia. They are likely to recur.

One day a thirty-year-old man came to see me in my clinic. He had moved from the south of England to Rotherham on account of his job. He had a history of allergy occurring all year round, suggesting his sensitivity was due to house dust mites as well as pollen. Over the years, he had undergone repeated removal of his polyps both in the south of England

and near his new home in Yorkshire. He was treated by his GP with antihistamine tablets and a nasal steroid spray with no success.

I could see he had polyps which needed surgery again. I listened as he said: "I wake up in the middle of night with mucous in my throat and occasional headache. The watery discharge from my nose is worse from my right nostril and it gets much worse when I put my head down." I went over his history with him again, I then took a sample of the fluid streaming from his right nostril and sent it off for laboratory examination.

I made an appointment for him to return the following week. The result from the laboratory was as I expected. The clear fluid was cerebral-spinal fluid from the meninges covering his brain! I sent him for a scan and that showed the loss of some bone in the floor of his skull, opening into his right nasal cavity. The fluid surrounding and cushioning the brain was leaking through the hole in the floor of his skull and streaming down his right nostril. I referred him to a neurosurgeon who successfully repaired the cribriform plate in the floor of his skull.

It is worth mentioning that surgical damage to the cribriform plate is a known hazard when polys are pulled instead of dissected away. In severe cases, brain tissue can hang in the nasal cavity, presenting as polyps. All ENT surgeons are aware of this.

Nose bleeds are very common as an ENT emergency. Stella, a young lady of 16, came to my clinic accompanied by her mother. She complained of frequent nose bleeds. "She gets these nose bleeds," said her mother "and each time we go *again* to the local hospital."

"Yes," said Stella "I'm getting *really* fed up with it!"

133

I asked: "What do they do when you go to the hospital?"

"Ah," said Stella, "It's awful. First, they put a piece of gauze in my nose and spray some local anaesthetic on the gauze." Stella stopped to think. "Then they look up my nose to see where the blood is coming from, then they burn the bleeding point with an electric machine. It doesn't hurt because my nose is numb by that time. After that, they pack my nose with special ribbon gauze. It usually settles down after a few days, but sometimes the bleeding doesn't stop, and I have to go back *again*."

Stella's mother said: "We went to the GP and we said we're getting *nowhere* with Stella's nosebleeds, could we see a specialist? So here we are!"

I sent a blood sample off to check for any bleeding disorder and I checked her blood pressure. I sprayed some local anaesthetic into her nose and asked her to wait for few minutes for the anaesthetic to take effect. When Stella and her mum came back into my consulting room, I examined her nose with the endoscope and could see the past bleeding points demarcated by raw and red patches. I also checked her nose for any bony injury. During examination, her mum said: "Stella is fed up with nose bleeds every month for the last two years." Suddenly the penny dropped!

Stella probably had a condition called endometriosis, where the lining of the womb grows not only inside the womb but outside too, on internal organs and – in Stella's case – on the lining of her nose. During her monthly period, the tissue in her nose responded to the female hormones and shed itself, causing her nose to bleed. But now we had to prove it!

I admitted her for a general anaesthetic and took a sample of the tissue for analysis. Two days later I saw Stella again and told her and her mum the result of the biopsy. Sure

134

enough, the tissue that bled in Stella's nose every month *was* the same tissue that lines the womb and is sensitive to the same female hormones.

Sometimes reaching a medical diagnosis involves thinking outside the box, a good deal of detective work and – last but not least – some medical knowledge. We had unravelled the mystery! I referred Stella to a gynaecologist, and she prescribed hormonal treatment. It is well known that this condition can be present in a number of places in the body.

A thirty-year old man came to see me complaining of headache and frequent dizzy spells, particularly when he exercised. He had seen his GP, a physiotherapist and an osteopath on several occasions, all to no avail. The GP then sent him to a cardiac physician, who had skull X-rays taken and organised a heart tracing. As his symptoms were not severe, he carried on with his life and exercise routine. Fortunately, no abnormality was found in his head. He was told his dizziness was possibly stress-related and was advised relaxation.

His symptoms of dizziness continued, so eventually his GP referred him to the ENT department, and he was booked to see me. I listened carefully to everything he had to tell me. He was a shelf-packer in the large local supermarket. In his spare time, he loved to go to the gymnasium and was a keen bodybuilder. Interestingly, during our discussion, he mentioned that every time he stocked the top shelf in the supermarket or raised his arms above his head at the gym, his symptoms got worse. I sent him for a neck X-ray and asked for skull X-rays taken previously to be brought to my desk.

On his next consultation, I showed him his X-rays. I pointed out a cervical rib which should have been in his chest

135

– but was in his neck – and an abnormal calcified band of tissue on the other side of his neck. Both abnormalities had been present since birth.

I ordered a scan and nerve studies and then sought the cardiologist's opinion. I referred the patient to the chest surgeon who advised early surgery. This man had lived with the abnormality for so long and had come to no harm, but now we knew that fatal complications were a possibility. I arranged surgery in Sheffield, where, together with my chest surgeon colleague, we removed the rib on the one side and the fibrous band on the other.

18. The Visit

IN THE SPRING of 1979 Kate sent a letter off to my parents, saying we looked forward to the day when they would visit us in England. She invited them to "Stay with us for our spring and summer; it will be lovely to see you and the weather should be very pleasant." They wrote back that they would be delighted to come after the wedding of my youngest brother Ravi, that winter.

They arrived at Heathrow airport in 1980, during the lovely month of June. Louise, Paul, and I had gone to meet them whilst Kate stayed at home with thirteen-month-old Clare. Kate was now expecting our fourth child the following February.

We watched the tide of airline passengers stream through the exit gate. There was no sign of my parents, so we waited, and we waited. An hour later, two tiny figures emerged into the Arrivals Hall. "There they are!" I exclaimed. We rushed forward with arms open wide. "Oh! It's great to see you! Did you have a comfortable journey? You must be exhausted! Shall we have a cup of tea?" All my words came tumbling out at once.

"We're so glad to see *you*!" they said as they hugged me, then Louise and Paul. Over breakfast at an airport café, they explained that, on arrival, they had been escorted to the Medical Room for a physical examination, a chest X-Ray and to fill in a detailed medical questionnaire.

We collected the car, put their two small suitcases in the boot, and at last drove towards M1 North. Looking out the car window as the countryside sped by, my Mum said, "It's so green, so beautiful!"

"There's a lot of cars on the road, Sat. No bicycles?" said my Dad. "No, of course not." He corrected himself, "I've heard about these motorways. Very fast, aren't they?"

As we coursed along, Louise's head drooped onto my Mother's lap and she fell asleep. Paul, sensing a break in the conversation, said: "I've got a new bicycle." He informed his Grandfather: "It's a Grifter." My Dad nodded sagely, wondering if he should be pleased, surprised or shocked. "I've just come back from a school trip to North Yorkshire," Paul continued, "We stayed in a log cabin and slept in bunk beds." Again, Dad nodded and smiled. "We had beans and sausage for breakfast and a big boy tipped beans onto a junior's head."

"Ohh!" My Dad exclaimed.

"In the field, we played Frisbees with dried cow-pats," Paul's eyes shone fondly at the memory. "And when we went to bed," he said, warming to his subject, "The masters went out to the pub!"

Eventually the conversation lulled and all except me – the driver – dozed off. We swept into the driveway in the early afternoon. Kate and Clare were at the front door to meet us. Kate touched my parents' feet and then there was much hugging and kissing. We drank tea in the garden. The air was warm, and the sunshine was golden. Insects hummed and buzzed around our lush, green garden, as we sat in the dappled shade of the cherry-blossom tree. I was content.

Kate had already prepared a meal of spiced mixed vegetables, lentils, pilau rice and chapatis. We had a fresh mango dessert and more masala tea. "How pleasant it is to sit here, Sat, in this green oasis of yours" said my Dad, in his grammatically perfect, old-fashioned way of speaking. (Official business, Law Courts and University lectures use the English language in India, therefore no slang or fashionable modern phrases creep into the text or spoken word.) "The day we left" said Mum, "it was 38C! The temperature will climb higher each day until the Monsoon arrives in August."

Dad told the children: "Monsoon is the name we give to the seasonal rain that falls on the south in June and travels up to reach the north in August." He sat back in his garden chair and heaved a sigh, "It's so wonderful here. You've a good life, son," He then got up to go and pick raspberries from the raspberry canes in the orchard.

We chatted until the sun went down. My father spoke English and four other languages besides, but my mother spoke only Hindi. It was lovely conversing with her in my mother tongue. "I'm worried," she said in Hindi, "How will Ravi fetch the milk in the morning? He's never done it before."

I laughed and said: "He's a big boy now, Mum, he's 26 and married. I'm sure he'll be able to work that one out."

I heard the latest news of my family, the neighbours and all the goings-on in the street. After early dinner, my parents settled down in their bedroom for the night.

Early next morning, Kate passed my parents' bedroom and popped her head round the door. "Are you alright? May I get you anything?" she enquired.

"Yes, yes, we are really fine," said Dad. And those were the last words he spoke before he was struck down and found *he could not speak at all*.

At about 6.30am, Mum called: "Sat! Sat! Come quick!" As I rushed into the room, Dad lay in bed, whilst Mum hovered over him.

"Are you alright?" I asked him, but he could not answer. I reached over and held both his hands. He grasped me tight with his left hand, but his right hand hung limp on the coverlet. I knew that he had suffered a stroke. A blood vessel had burst and was bleeding into the left side of his brain. He needed urgent hospital admission. I rang a hospital colleague, then we bundled Dad into the car and took him to hospital. He was admitted to a ward and I waited in the day room. Eventually my colleague entered the room.

"You know, Sat, don't you?" he began as he took a seat beside me.

"Yes, he's had a stroke."

He gazed at me earnestly and said: "He's had a major heart attack followed by a left- sided brain haemorrhage."

Dad stayed in the hospital for ten weeks. Mum and I visited every day. He had physiotherapy, speech therapy and the most wonderful nursing care. Eventually, my colleague declared Dad had reached a plateau and the muscle weakness on the right side of his body would always require him to walk with a walking frame; his slurred speech, memory loss and depression would also improve no further. So we brought him home, a changed man, but nevertheless alive. And for that, we were deeply grateful.

Dad and Mum had been so much looking forward to their visit to us in England. We all did feel sorry for them but could not change the situation. During Dad's stay in hospital, Mum spent her early mornings sitting on the sofa, wrapped in her shawl, praying. The visit they had dreamed of had gone so horribly wrong. She had planned to have her hair fashionably cut, wear western clothes, and visit a pub. Prior to leaving for England, she told her friends and neighbours that she would come back looking very different.

Clare, our small daughter, seemed to sense her Grandma's loneliness, so wherever my Mum went, Clare went too. Clare would not eat unless she was sitting on my Mum's knee; she wanted Grandma at bedtime, and they spent long summer afternoons swinging together on the garden swing-seat. Every evening, Mum and I visited Dad in the hospital.

We took Mum to a Cash and Carry supermarket. She looked down the aisles stretching away into the distance, goods piled on either side "I never knew there were such places. I'm punch-drunk with it all, Sat!" she said.

"You buy whatever you like, Mum," I said, "It'll do you good to have a bit of fun, don't worry about the paying bit." So, Mum piled fleece bed throws, quilted jackets, kitchen blenders and toys into her trolley, typically none of these were for her.

"I'd love to go to the seaside," Mum said one crisp autumn day, "My Father took me to see the sea when we lived in Karachi."

"What age were you when you went to the seaside?" Louise asked. I translated to Mum, and she replied: "I don't know, Louise, I suppose I would have been about your age." Louise thought not knowing your age was thrilling! But, on the other hand, what about birthday presents and cake?

The next fine day, we loaded the car up and set off for Scarborough and Whitby. It was great to see Mum relaxing and enjoying herself with the family. "I'd like to experience a typically English day at the sea-side," she said, so we had shrimps and ice cream on the beach. We paddled in the sea and walked along the promenade. We spotted a fish and chip café, half-timbered mock-Tudor on the outside, very crowded and very warm on the inside. The tables were covered with gingham tablecloths; waitresses in white pinafores brought pots of tea and piles of buttered bread to the tables. The plates of battered fish and chips emerging from the kitchen were towering creations of golden crispness. Mum said she could live on fish, chips and peas for the rest of her life.

141

We had visited Blackpool Illuminations every year since we came to live in Yorkshire, and we made the visit that year with Mum. The children were in their element on the amusement rides and the slot machine arcades. Mum was delighted by the illuminations and the crowds of jolly people.

As my parents had been keen to see London, I took Mum, Louise, and Paul for a long weekend. We visited Buckingham Palace, Madam Tussaud, the Houses of Parliament; and, of course, we went shopping. Hamley's, the largest toy shop in the world, was on the list. "I'll buy a gift for all our grand-children. Now let's see, that's five boys and five girls." And she headed off into the stream of shoppers. She was a woman on a mission.

My parents knew that public houses were a way of life over here, and Mum decided it was a good way to see the British at play. I took her to our local pub, and we chatted over drinks. She was delighted to be sitting next to a group of young women out on their own. "Wonderfully modern and thoroughly liberated," she pronounced them in Hindi.

She was on top form that night, as, on our return home, she swayed towards Kate and gave a good impression of having drunk a few pints, when, in fact she had half a pint of lemonade and a packet of cheese and onion crisps.

"Would you like to come grocery shopping with me?" Kate asked and Mum agreed. The Asian corner shop was nearby; its shelves were stacked from floor to ceiling with everything an Asian customer could want. And, if by chance they did not have it, they would get it for you.

Mum eyed the tall man behind the counter and he leaned forward to see my mother more clearly. Kate introduced them and the proprietor's face lit up. "Mataji, you are Mrs Mehta's mother-in-law?"

142

She replied in Hindi: "Haan," (yes) then she said, again in Hindi: "I really think I have seen you before, but I can't think where it was." He leaned further and in a conspiratorial voice said: "Did you ever live in Kamalia in Lyallpur District before Partition?" He was recalling events from 34 years ago, when he would have been about twelve years of age. "Did you have the really big farm near the railway station?"

My mother's eyes widened, and she nodded. The proprietor clapped his hands and exclaimed: "I remember you, Mataji!"

My mother looked faint and a chair was brought so she could sit down whilst she murmured: "Oh! I can't believe it! Six thousand miles I've come, and I meet someone from home!"

We put a glass of water in her hand as she said: "Yes, you were a little boy last time I saw you." Her voice dropped to a whisper as she said: "Tell me, what happened to our farm and the house after we left?"

He looked sober and replied: "Aah, the farm was divided up. A land-grab, you might say. The house was ransacked, not one door left on its hinges and then it was set on fire."

"That farm," she said, between sips of water, "the land and the five houses had been in the Mehta family for as long as anyone can remember. My husband's father could trace the farm back three hundred years!"

He saw how upset my mother was. He said: "The houses have been rebuilt and, as they were big houses, they are government offices now."

My mother visited the Asian corner shop often after that and, whilst Kate went round with her trolley selecting her purchases, Mum sat and chatted with the shopkeeper asking after her old friends and neighbours.

Mum sat on the chair whilst the shopkeeper listened. She recalled the house, surrounded by the mobs, fiery torches blazing; she recalled the screams and shouts, the crack of firearms and the clash of swords. Tears came to her eyes as she recounted the slaughter of her brother- in-law. "That was the worse time of my life."

I truly believe that the shopkeeper's quiet and sympathetic ear was, for Mum, a therapy beyond price.

19. Travels

A HOLIDAY like no other began with a telephone interview.

The Ox-Venture Experiment (not advertised as a holiday) was a trekking holiday to Nepal. "You'd really enjoy it!" said Clare our daughter, who had been the previous year. The Experiment was conducted by a very lively ex-SAS officer. One group climbed to first base camp at 17,000 feet, and our group would trek to 9,000 feet, sail the rapids of the Karnali River and go on a Jungle Safari. Our group was open to all ages and abilities, including the physically disabled. The idea being that the able-bodied help the disabled. There was only one rule, made clear in the interview: "*grumblers need not apply.*"

We met the retired officer at a pub near Newbury for a briefing, "Right! Listen Up!" he said, "a minimal amount of clothes, everything has to go in a rucksack." He suggested to train for the trip we run up and down stairs fifty times a day. He said his sponsorship of a school and an orphanage were partially funded by the holidays he arranged. Our group was made up of a Leader, a Medical Doctor, a Nurse, and two of each age group, ranging from 20 to 60 years old. Some of us were physically fit and some were disabled.

Kate and I did not volunteer as medics, we just wanted a holiday. But our leader suggested that, as I could speak Hindi which is very like Nepalese, we could help local villagers as we ascended the mountain side. He added with a twinkle in his eye: "And they've already heard you're coming." So we went home, discarded some clothes out of our rucksack and packed some medical supplies.

Kathmandu Airport is over 4,000 feet in altitude and the runways are approached through a narrow gap in the mountains. The plane circled three times before making its final approach. On the banks of the Bagmati river in Kathmandu town, funeral pyres smouldered, monks meditated, and little boys dived from the narrow bridge into the water. The place was alive with monkeys, goats, chickens and parakeets. On the high street, a shop called *Wet Dreams* hired out river canoes.

Leaving Kathmandu the following day, we bounced along the road through thick green jungle. Deer, wild pigs, snakes and tigers lived in the forest. The rain came down in torrents, so that night, rather than try to pitch tents, we stayed in a village.

We arrived after dark. The night sky was studded with stars like thousands of diamonds. We picked our way in the velvet blackness along the mud road and stepped over the dead dog in the middle of the pathway. We found our way to the village school where we were to stay the night. The women of our party slept in the classrooms and men slept on the floor in the corridors: *"grumblers need not apply"* came to mind.

In the blackness Kate saw sets of shining eyes creeping down the wall towards where our friend Vicky slumbered peacefully. Outside were screeching noises and inside scratching noises, a symphony of nocturnal wildlife, near and very much alive. Kate woke to find her pillow chewed to shreds and her hair wet. "Ah," said Jack, a fellow traveller "rats ran over me last night and under your door!"

The following morning the rain had stopped. We thanked the village for their kindness and hospitality in our hour of need and headed for the river. At the end of the day, I suggested to Kate that she wash her hair in the river before we pitched the tent. It was the first night we had no access to electricity, so we ate by firelight and undressed by torchlight. Kate and

I enjoyed looking up at the night sky and the outline of distant mountain peaks, pale in the light of the moon. We went to sleep listening to the water lapping on the riverbank.

"Coo-ee! Coo-ee! Hellooo Uncle Doctor, you awake, Uncle you in there?" Our tent flap lifted as a cheery little face looked in to tell us a queue was gathering outside to have free medical consultations. "Subha-prabhata, good morning" the children said as we emerged into the bright morning sunlight. It was 6am. "Eating, you please, we wait." The villagers *had* heard that a Hindi speaking Doctor would be amongst the party and would be happy to hold a clinic for anyone who needed medical advice and medication.

The consultations were very public, as the villagers gathered round and looked on. They managed the queue and made sure no one was left out. Patient after patient laid on the ground, in the middle of our circle of tents. "Tell him about your belly ache, Grandma!" they encouraged the elderly lady stretched out on the ground, "and you're itching!" I made a diagnosis of intestinal worms and gave her some anthelmintic tablets. When a mountain guide came forward for examination, the collective advice was: "Tell him about you getting thinner and thinner!" I palpated his lymph glands, and they were enlarged so I advised he and his family go to Pokhara for chest X-Rays. And so, the morning went on, until the last patient was seen. Tropical and third world medicine is very different from anything either our group Doctor or Nurse would have come across in their training.

"We'll give you a hand, just tell us what to do!" said our willing fellow travellers. So, no medical experience required, they shampooed little heads full of lice and nits.

As we trekked along one day, we came upon a group of women sitting on a dry-stone wall in the morning

147

sunshine, waiting for us. I don't know how they knew we were on our way up, but there they were. One of them, had a large bandage round her foot and she asked me to have a look. She said she had stepped on a long rusty nail a week ago and had a deep and penetrating wound on the sole of her foot. She had travelled down the mountain to a dispensary and been treated there. The wound was so expertly packed with iodine-soaked ribbon gauze that I left it in place and bandaged her foot up again. She then produced a syringe, needle and a phial of Penicillin. "They gave me a Penicillin and Anti-Tetanus injection at the dispensary," she said, "this is my second dose. Will you give me?" I was very impressed with the treatment she had received.

Listening to my patients in their own language was a big advantage. I had brought with me a battery-powered head torch, a pair of fine crocodile forceps, a few syringes and I had been collecting medicine from the hospital pharmacy, surgical equipment and dressings too, so I had come very well equipped. In one mountainside clinic, I saw a lady who unmistakably had advanced tuberculosis: she had chest symptoms, night sweats and tuberculous abdominal lymph glands. I advised that she and her whole family refer themselves, as an emergency, to the main hospital in Kathmandu. I understand Nepalese well, so my patients could speak to me freely, which made my diagnosis faster and more accurate and my instructions to the patient more easily understood.

On the Karnali river we shot the rapids and rode the white water. I was assigned to help a woman in our group of travellers, paralysed from the waist down and confined to a wheelchair. Kate had a young man with a neurological disorder to keep safe. In the canoe, Kate snuggled him into a beanbag and secured the large Velcro straps. "There's only one way he's going to get out of *that.*" She thought "if we hit a rock!" And that is what happened – they hit a rock! He flew straight up into the air and landed in the river, a few feet from their boat. The current was strong and fast, Kate held him fast with an oar, but he let it go and slid rapidly downstream with the current. Kate thought: *I've lost him! He can't use his legs! he'll drown and wash up dead somewhere!* but the strong arms of our Leader caught him, and he was restored back into his beanbag, grinning and exhilarated by his near-death adventure. He was just disappointed that no-one had recorded the event on camera.

"What's for dinner?" we asked when we finally pulled up onto the riverbank. "Chicken" came the reply. Our lovely Sherpas then ran after the chicken and wrung its neck. We spent a magical evening round the campfire, steaming in our drying clothes and singing half-forgotten childhood songs, until one by one, we drifted off to bed.

The following day, after travelling further down the river, we hauled our canoes up on the river bank by a very remote village. The village was surrounded by marijuana, a weed growing lush and abundant as high as a child's head. The Ox-Venture Organiser had given us dire warnings at our initial briefing: "Don't touch it, even a leaf left in a trouser pocket, wilted and forgotten *will* be detected at the airport by sniffer dogs." He added: "I will not be bailing you out of jail. And – boy! – you *don't* want to see the inside of a Nepalese jail!" Most of the villagers were happily stoned; men and women stuffed clay pipes with weed and sat around in a daze.

Two ladies had sidled up, one on each side of me. They were steering me towards a rickety bamboo ladder set against the mud brick wall of a house. Clearly, they wanted me to climb the ladder to their bedroom. The bedroom had only three walls. "Kate," said Vicky, "that's your husband there, don't you think we ought to go and rescue him?"

"No, he's having fun. Anyway," Kate observed as the ladies turned to smile at us, "I don't think he's too keen, they've only got one tooth between them!"

A potter made vessels of all shapes and sizes, and his pots were in great demand as everything, food, clothes, even babies were kept, suspended above the ground in the clay pots, on account of the river rats.

As we travelled through the jungle, thousands of insects and leeches clung to us. I had them, big, black and squirming, sucking firmly on my back, my shoulder, my legs and another stuck to my cap. I had experienced leeches in Australia, where I had attracted about 200 tiny squirming leeches; on that occasion Kate had rubbed me with salt, put me in a warm shower and handed me a large whisky, in that order. Nepalese leeches, by contrast, are so large they look as if they could drain you of blood in half an hour. For some reason they seem afraid to bite Kate.

Ever onwards and upwards, we reached our camp as darkness descended, pitching the tents by torchlight. The nocturnal rustles, snorts and squeals in the vegetation that surrounded the camp were thrilling. Millions of fireflies flitted their tiny lights from bush to bush and I could not resist my boyhood prank: I dived into the bushes, caught dozens of these little fellas and put them under my shirt. When I sprang from the vegetation, eerily aglow, our travelling companions shrieked, "Aaah! What's that? You nearly gave me a heart attack! I thought you were a ghost!"

We went to bed contented and tired, mindful that the rustles and snorts around us had always been here, we were guests in *animal* territory now, untamed and sparsely inhabited by humans.

In the morning, as the sun rose, it became clear why we came here in the dark. We opened the tent flap and there, rising majestically before us was the snow-covered Annapurna mountain range, bathed in red and gold. Machapuchare (Fishtail Mountain) rose in the centre to a height of nearly 23,000 feet. The early morning clouds were below us, resting on the valley floor, even the birds flew below. Everest looked so close and so clear.

Breakfast at 9,000 feet was porridge, wild honey and boiled-up tea overlooking and the most spectacular view in the world. We will never see its like again.

The Limbu, Rai and Kirat people, the original inhabitants of the Kathmandu Valley, welcomed us into their village. They carried Kukri knives in their belts and wore woven Dhaka fabric in brightly coloured patterns. These are the people from which the Gurkha Regiments in the British Army come. There was hardly a house which did not have an army connection.

That night on the mountainside was party night and also it was Vicky's birthday. We bought some locally made alcohol for the party. It came in interesting containers: a two-gallon watering can, a kettle and a plastic bucket. The cook made a chocolate birthday cake. In the centre of the cake was one large white candle, dripping with wax. That cake, baked right under the shadow of Everest (or Chomolungma if you are in Tibet, and Sagarmatha if you are in Nepal) tasted better than any before or since, even though it tasted of curried chocolate.

On our descent we heard a pitiful wail from the forest behind us. An animal hurt, I thought. I followed the sound and there, in the forest glade stood a little boy about four years old, bawling at the top of his voice, tears and snot streaming down his face; "I don't know where I AM!" he

151

bawled in Nepalese, in my ear. "I'm LOST!!" his voice rose to a crescendo, "Where's my BROTHER?"

I squatted down and said in Hindi: "Put your arms round my neck and climb on my back." He put his trust in me and did as I told him. With him snivelling snot onto my head, we descended the hillside together, and made for the village below. He and his big brother had come up with other children from the village to see us, and he had become separated and left behind. In the village, his brother was frantic, neighbours and friends scurried hither and thither, searching the village, and his parents were out combing the surrounding fields. Beaming with relief but still snivelling onto my head, he gave a shout of joy when he spotted his big brother. He wriggled down from my shoulders and, without a backward glance, ran into his brother's embrace.

When the time came to go home, we were crestfallen. "I never want to sleep in a bed again." Kate remarked. I thought we had been through so much together, shared so many experiences together, that we had become like a family. The Ox-Venture Experiment was a resounding success. The ex-SAS Officer arranged a reunion at the pub where our adventure had begun. After dinner, Kate recited her poem, *The Dream Team*, about the most unlikely set of trekkers ever.

We sat in the garden with seven of our friends one summer evening. We had worked hard all afternoon putting up three huge marquees on the lawn in readiness for the Parishes' forthcoming Plant Fayre to be held in our garden. The evening was warm as the sun sank in the West. A golden glow bathed the garden in long shadows. We sat and drank chilled beer. We were pleasantly mellow as the conversation turned to other Parish events.

"What's the Jumbulance like then, Ian?" I asked. The Jumbulance bus was the vehicle that would carry us from Wakefield to Lourdes, the well-known Pilgrimage town in France. The organisers were asking for volunteer doctors, nurses and helpers to go. Kate and I wanted to volunteer but needed to know what to expect. We had been organising plant sales, barbecues and coffee mornings in our houses to raise funds to provide the very sick and their relatives too with financial help to make the trip.

I wanted to know what a trip to Lourdes was like. A member of our Parish organised a Pilgrimage every second year, taking the seriously sick and infirm in a specially converted coach, to France. The coach is equipped with beds, kitchen, toilet and reclining seats. "Well," said Ian, "Let's put it this way, as *you* would be Crew, your needs will come *last*." He grinned. "Picture this: we're hurtling down a motorway in France, it's three o'clock in the morning and old Bill, who's paralysed down one side, says: *Quick! I feel sick!*" Ian knew he had our undivided attention now. He warmed to the subject and took a long draught of his beer, "so I manage to grab a sick bowl and shuffle old Bill to the toilet in the bus, which is, as you can imagine, about five feet square, I'm holding Bill up over my shoulder while he's being sick and then he says, Ian! I've got the runs! so I've got one hand with a wodge of toilet paper on his bum and the other holding the sick bowl over my shoulder, while we swerve to left and right along the motorway!" he grinned, "But don't let that put you off going, it's a great experience!"

I signed up.

The group I went with was made up of two priests, a group Leader, three nurses, a medic and a number of helpers. We referred to our disabled as our VIPs. We had three people in wheelchairs and one on a stretcher. We had a person who had a heart-lung transplant and he'd also had a

153

mild stroke. Kate and I went to visit all those joining us on this trip. I checked the medication and the medical conditions of each traveller.

The journey by road and ferry takes around twenty-six hours. "Bye, safe journey!" and "Say one for me!" and "Ring when you get there!" shouted the parishioners, friends and families as the buses pulled away. Our excitement was palpable, but soon eyes began to close and heads began to droop. A serene calm descended as we sped towards the ferry in Dover.

We were then onto French soil and Lourdes would be reached in five hours – but first a stop for breakfast, a coffee and a cognac to celebrate our safe arrival.

Our destination hotel was purpose built. The Grotto, where it all started in 1858, is a cave on the banks of the River Gave where a poor peasant girl, Bernadette Soubirous, saw several apparitions of a Lady. When Bernadette asked "Who are you?" the Lady replied: "I am the Immaculate Conception."

People knew that poor uneducated Bernadette could not have made that up. The Lady asked Bernadette to scratch in the ground, and bystanders thought: "Ah, the poor child has gone mad." But a spring of water welled up and has flowed ever since. Many miraculous cures have been attributed to the healing waters. I saw faith in action, everyone helping everyone else with a smile. Wheelchairs ruled the pathways and restaurants cleared spaces for trolleys. This was love and faith I had not seen before and I was very impressed.

The Torchlight Procession at dusk with the voices of thousands of pilgrims, young and old, able bodied and disabled, from all corners of the world singing "Ave, ave, ave, Maria," was one of the highlights of the trip.

Back at the hotel we had evenings filled with song, dance and bingo sessions. The most seriously ill, who were weary and wanted to do no more than rest, were helped into bed.

On a picnic the following day, we overlooked a lake and saw the Pyrenees mountains in the background, a perfect spot to relax and unwind. It became apparent that a change in the group dynamics was taking place. The help was not all in the one direction.

"Hey, want me to carry those coats?" said a wheelchair bound pilgrim; and also "Let me take the videos, I'll not be moving very far from here. You run across the meadow, like Maria in *The Sound of Music*, and I'll film it!" offered another person in a wheelchair. I silently applauded our VIPs, as we called our disabled comrades, who lent a listening ear to helpers' worries and troubles.

The last night was party night, with an amateur cabaret afterwards. Gerry's act was the one that brought the house down. Gerry was a large and jolly man. But on party night he transformed into Shirley Bassey. He burst onto the stage in a wig and a glittering sequinned gown. He sang 'Hey, big spender!" with more feeling and gusto than Shirley herself.

One of the Nurses and I did a duet: "Oh Doctor I'm in Trouble," she sang as she batted her eyelashes at the audience.

"Well Goodness Gracious Me," I crooned, although Peter Sellers does a better Indian accent than I...or is it me?

Kate went as a nurse the following year. She said on her return: "As we travelled home, I looked down the bus and it was clear that the group we brought back home was a very different group to the one we brought out.

"We were a family, we had enabled each other, we had come together and enjoyed a spiritual and social experience. This is the everyday miracle performed by Lourdes. No miraculous cures for our group of pilgrims this time, but a renewal of Faith and Hope like I have never seen!"

I went as a doctor the following year and then Kate and I went together. The group joined up with a neighbouring parish and became a jolly jamboree with singers and entertainers. Soon afterwards the trips ceased altogether.

20. Kate's Dad Goes to India Too

FIVE YEARS AFTER my parents' visit to England, I took Kate's Dad Tony to India.

In the summer of 1985, he was living in Quadring, Lincolnshire. Kate's mother had died back in April of that year and he was now living on his own, cooking for himself and remaining his usual cheerful self. My own father had also died in the month of May and I was going to visit my mother that winter.

"See if Dad would like to come with you," said Kate, "He'll say no, but we can ask..." To our surprise, the answer was: "Yes, I'd love to come!"

Tony, my father-in-law, was a typical English Gentleman: courteous, true to his word and upstanding in society, in manners and style. He was always smartly dressed in a suit on Sundays, and on weekdays a tweed jacket. Polished shoes were a must, unless he was in his Wellingtons, and he always wore a tie. He loved going for walks with the family. He was a keen gardener and very knowledgeable about farming and country life. He had not been out of the country since his days in the RAF, did not like Indian food and detested even a whiff of garlic; but it was one of the most interesting and pleasurable trips we ever made together.

I arranged the flights and informed my mother that I was bringing him with me. She wrote a personal letter to him, inviting him as her guest.

In those days, international flights started at mid-day in London and landed very early the next day in India. We arrived at the old Palam Airport, New Delhi, before Indira Gandhi Airport was built. As I have already written, the airport was a concrete construction like a large warehouse.

157

Fluorescent tube lighting shone with a harsh light; pigeons flew about, perching in the rafters above the ceiling fans. Officials in khaki, their berets worn military style, were everywhere.

Tony, or Dad as I now called him, was quite intrigued and surprised to see so many women employed at the airport. He said to me: "I'm used to seeing Indian women gliding along in silk saris, not in khaki uniform, what's all this?" and he waved his hand airily.

"These are women with power, and nobody messes with them," I said, "They're athletic and could pack a punch if needed."

He looked amused. We waited in the queue for ten minutes for visa and passport checks but, as I had a father-in-law from England, I was given preferential treatment and we passed through quite quickly.

In baggage reclaim, slumbering porters and long-haul passengers lay on the floor in a heap of luggage. The baggage collection machine was broken so all the baggage had to be brought through by hand.

My cousin Raj, wrapped up against the chill early morning air in an enormous cream shawl, came to collect us from the airport. Auto-rickshaws revved their little two-stroke engines, making a furious noise and emitting clouds of diesel fumes. The air was thick with smog as we came out of the airport and it hung over Delhi in a choking grey cloud until the thermals blew it away with the sunrise.

Raj was tall, statuesque, and friendly, always ready to chuckle. Tony said later, "I couldn't get over him; he was full of beans even at that time in the morning!" Raj's wife Vimal was up and waiting to greet us. It was five o'clock in the morning. As we sat at the breakfast table, Dad was flanked on either side by Raj and Vimal's children, Gautam and Neetu, who were about twelve and fourteen years old.

"Tell us about your family" said Neetu.

"Uncle Tony" said Gautam, "you're a sort of farmer, are you? Outside even when it rains?"

"Thinking of rain," said Neetu "In cricket in England, how is it that rain stops play one minute, and then in ten minutes the rain stops and they're back playing?"

"In India," said Gautam, "when it rains, it lasts for weeks."

Neetu then gently put out her hand to rest on Dad's and said: "We were sorry to hear about the loss of Aunty last year."

Dad's heart was touched that these two youngsters should be so sensitive to his loss. He thanked them for their thoughts and gave details of his job, managing forty acres of glasshouse, producing hundreds of thousands of plants for well-known supermarkets in the UK. He enjoyed this lively early morning conversation and recalled their company with pleasure, on many occasions when back in England.

We rested before taking the last leg of our journey to Meerut. The Sikh taxi driver wore a magnificent saffron coloured turban and had pictures of Guru Nanak on the dashboard. He greeted us with a great smile and then drove with great skill and at a cracking pace through the streets of Delhi.

"Whole families crammed onto one scooter, husband wife and two children!" marvelled Dad as we sped through the morning rush hour. Many smiled and waved to us.

"We're out of Delhi now, Dad, on the Grand Trunk Road, heading north," I said.

The traffic thinned and became more rural. Three-wheeled minibuses chugged along carrying twelve to fifteen people. We passed highly decorated lorries, garlanded, and painted, like traditional *vardos* (gypsy caravans). Halfway,

159

we stopped at a small village. Dad was interested to see exotic fruits and vegetables piled high on the carts. "I have never come across custard apples or starfruit and I've never even heard of black lotus roots or okra." He saw roasted corn on the cob and sugar-cane juice.

Suddenly there was a commotion and a minor political leader, visiting the village, was announced repeatedly over a crackling loudspeaker. We saw his garlanded figure swaggering along the little market square, so we decided it was time to continue on our way.

By mid-morning, two hours later, we had reached our destination. The house is at the end of a cul- de-sac, too narrow for the taxi to drive down, so we parked in the lane, unloaded the luggage, and walked towards the small figure of my beloved Mother. As usual, she had been waiting for us since dawn. She was standing in the middle of the path in a white sari (the colour of mourning in India) with a brown woollen shawl over her head and shoulders. I bent forward and touched Mother's feet in a gesture of respect, and she opened her arms and gave me a big hug.

She was very keen to greet my father-in-law. She shook his hand and said: "Hello, Tony, you are very, very, welcome, stay with us as long as you wish." She added: "It is my turn to welcome you, as you welcomed me to England five years ago." She had visited Kate's parents in Lincolnshire when she was in England.

It appeared all the neighbours knew that we were coming on that day, as many were at their garden gates watching. The children in the path stopped playing, curious to see us.

Dad and I were greeted by my brothers Kuckoo and his wife Sneh, and Ravi and his wife Reena; they had taken a day off from the office to greet us. Mother had given strict instructions and advised her daughters-in-law regarding what Tony could and could not eat. They made us an omelette and toasted bread.

We retired to the flat roof and veranda on the first floor. We had two bedrooms and a bathroom. It was a quiet retreat up there; we could see all around the houses as well as the sky full of kites. In my boyhood I had been a champion kite flyer, and to see them fluttering in the blue sky evoked distant memories of carefree days. Indeed, kite-flying had been my favourite hobby, jumping from one roof to the other in pursuit of a kite.

Back to my journey with my Father-in-law: in the evening, we dined on roast chicken, specially prepared for him. My sisters-in-law were very good at adapting to the English way of cooking. We sat for a while on the veranda, before bed; the night sky was velvety black and studded with millions of stars. We spent relaxing days and restful nights at home in Meerut.

In the early morning there was the familiar cry of the vegetable seller in the street below, rumbling along with his hand cart. Some things never change: he still had spinach, piled high, and white radishes, still draped with wet hessian sacking. He kept the mound of fresh vegetables from wilting in the sunshine with the frequent sprinkling of water. There was still the tup, tup, tup, of laundry being slapped and beaten on the flat stone floor downstairs.

But my Mother no longer climbed the stairs nowadays, so my sister-in-law brought the morning tea up to our room. The bathroom had a small sink and a mirror. Water was fetched in a bucket from the tap on the veranda, topped up with hot water from the kettle. There was a cake of red soap, cut from a large slab, the very perfume of which reminded me of my childhood. Dad smiled and recalled: "I used it during the Second World War in Egypt."

161

My Father-in-law was my Mother's guest, so dozens of visitors were constantly arriving at the house just to come to meet him and invite him for dinner or other social functions. Kuckoo and Ravi arranged for us to visit interesting places. The Military Dairy Farm was of special interest as Dad was a horticulturalist and involved with plants and animals in England,: he was very interested in the everyday activities on the farm and the bottling plant.

We were invited to a very special rooftop garden. The plants were of different varieties to the plants my father-in-law grew in England. The gardeners told him how the plants survived temperatures of 45C and unremitting sunshine. He was impressed by the fact that they sowed seeds collected from the year before. They had no hybrid or grafted plants. Most of the flowers were highly scented: fragrant roses, lantana, jasmine, marigold, snapdragon, delphinium, petunia and hibiscus bloomed everywhere. In particular, Dad liked the fragrant tuberose.

One day we took a rickshaw and spent half the day wandering in the Meerut Military Cantonment, formerly known as Company Bagh, but now Gandhi Park. The area covered several acres and boasted a great variety of flora and fauna new to him, such as banyan trees, their roots like twisted ropes; bougainvillea, scrambling over walls in a riot of red, orange and hot pink; and neem trees, known for their antiseptic properties (if the ends of a twig are chewed, it makes a reasonable toothbrush). The lawns were well tended and extended to several playing fields and cricket pitches. The thwack of willow on leather could be heard there from dawn until dusk.

"In this garden," I told Dad, "I spent my teenage years, studying in the shade of these ashoka, mango, tamarind and peepal trees." There was a group of girls

162

having a picnic; on seeing Dad, they came across and we spent a half-hour talking about England.

Just before this visit to India, I had seen a patient in my consulting rooms who greeted me with "Namaste!" (Hello in Hindi.) He then told me that from 1920 to 1930 he had been in India in the army and how much he had enjoyed his stay and adventures. I asked him where he had spent his time. He answered: "Most of it in the north of India." I told him I came from the North of India and I was going the following week to visit my Mother in Meerut. He was amazed and said: "I was posted in the Meerut Cantonment and had a wonderful time there. Would you take some photos of Meerut Railway Station and Meerut Cantonment Parade Ground?"

Whilst playing polo on the Maidan (Parade Ground) he had been thrown from his horse and sustained a fractured skull. After many weeks recovering, he had been appointed clerk to the Regimental Chaplain at St John's Church in Meerut Cantonment. His duty in the vestry each morning was to type letters and prepare accounts. One morning the Chaplain asked if the cupboards could be cleaned out, and piles of books, registers and documents were taken out to allow the caretaker to wash the shelves. My patient looked through some old records and was able to read of the day that the Indian Mutiny started. "At ten minutes to four, on the afternoon of 10th May 1857," he said, "the first cannon shell to be fired hit the clock of St John's Church and stopped it at precisely the time and date of the start of the 90-year struggle for Independence for India!"

Dad and I visited St John's Church. We found it half hidden under the shade of overgrown trees. Lichen covered gravestones that lay in disarray, hidden by the tall grasses. Creeping vines covered the stone walls and scrambled in profusion over tiny lead-paned windows. The gravestones told of whole families – men, women, and children from the British Garrison – who had succumbed to typhoid, malaria, or tuberculosis. A hand-drawn bier, with bicycle wheels stood under a tree. It had been used to transport coffins, but now lay forgotten and half hidden in the grass.

We pushed open the huge door and stepped into the dark interior of the Church. Inside, under a layer of dust, was an old piano. We opened the lid, blew years of dust from the black and ivory keys and struck a few notes; the piano was in tune. Hymn books were stacked at the end of the pews, near the slots in which the soldiers propped their rifles whilst attending services. On the walls, faded sepia photographs of soldiers in full military dress and topees gazed out, possibly for the last 130 years. A thick layer of dust and cobwebs lay on every surface. All was now quiet and fossilized in time.

Kuckoo arranged transport to go to Sardhana, fifteen miles from Meerut. Long ago a princess of the Muslim faith converted to Christianity and built a Cathedral at Sardhana. The Italian priest allowed us to view the church treasures, not normally shown to anyone, a special privilege for my Catholic Father-in-law. The little village that grew up near the Cathedral is a step back in time. The mud and cow-dung dwellings had low walls enclosing a courtyard. One end of the courtyard, a single windowless room with thatched roof, provided for sleeping, and at the other end a washroom and a latrine, the traditional rural dwelling in India.

Dad and I walked through the village followed by a crowd of unruly children. We could sometimes see the glint of a gold nose ring in the dark interior of the houses as a woman looked up from her chores. The children wanted to show us an old man weaving cloth on a wooden loom. His feet rocked back and forth as his shuttle flew backwards and forwards.

164

That evening, we visited my friend Kawal Loria, the doctor and family friend who had permitted me to sit in on his clinics when I was a medical student. "Let's have a drink at The Wheeler Club!" he exclaimed. The Club, in the Military Cantonment, was established during the British Raj. It had a driveway lined with mango and papaya trees and looked over a sweep of manicured lawns. The fiery blossoms of bougainvillea climbed over the doorway and bearers wearing white gloves served drinks in the bar.

Dad and I ordered a long cool beer. But the bearer thought pink gins, some Indian tonic water, and a tray of samosa and pakora snacks was a far more fitting sundowner for the English gentleman so that is what he brought for all of us. The manager of the club heard of Dad's arrival and came over to invite us to see artefacts of "The *real* Wheeler Club," as he put it, "in its Victorian hey-day." There were pictures of army officers with handlebar moustaches riding polo ponies. We saw the Regimental silver trophies and cut-glass decanters in glass cabinets and tiger skins and sabres on the walls. There was an impressive dining room and a large Billiards Room.

After spending a week with my mother in Meerut, we took leave, went by taxi to Delhi, and arrived at the Imperial Hotel on Connaught Place. It was in this hotel that Pandit Nehru, Mahatma Gandhi, Mohammad Ali Jinnah and Lord Mountbatten met to discuss the end of 200 years of British Rule.

Here also the plans were drawn up for the creation of Pakistan, demanded by Mohammed Ali Jinnah and agreed by Lord Mountbatten. The hotel has an extensive collection of colonial and post-colonial photographs and artefacts in a museum.

We were given a huge twin-bedded double room. We looked out from the window onto the hotel's private lawn where breakfast and afternoon tea is served. There is always a choice of Western or Indian food.

After spending three days at the Imperial Hotel, we agreed that Dad should see the Taj Mahal. We went on the Shatabdi Express train, travelling directly from Delhi to Agra. We reserved our seat and settled back for an enjoyable ride. "Shoe-shine, sir? I give you wonderful shine!" a shoe shiner wanted to polish Dad's suede shoes. A while later he came back. "Taxi, I arrange for you, sir? Taxi- man show you all round Agra. Very, very good guide!" He said with a shake of his head. He disappeared down the train and we did not see him again.

I had an Indian lunch on the train, which Dad found to be quite an interesting experience, although he had bread and omelette. We stayed at the opulent Clarke Hotel and the next morning went to see the Taj Mahal. As soon as we came out of the hotel, beggars besieged us from all sides, asking for money. The contrast between the gold-plated inside and the abject poverty outside the hotel was something Dad found very upsetting.

At the Taj Mahal, we were given 'The Tour.' We were shown chisel marks in the marble and blank spaces in the decoration, where rubies, emeralds, pearls and gold, had been stolen and are missing to this day.

From Fatehpur Sikri and the Agra Fort there is a good view of the Taj Mahal. Shah Jehan, who had built the Taj Mahal in memory of his favourite wife Arjumand Banu Begum (Mumtaz Mahal) was imprisoned by his son Aurangzeb in Agra Fort – so he could gaze at, but never go to, the mausoleum for the rest of his life.

After visiting Agra, we decided to visit my brother in Jaipur, Rajasthan. At the airport there was a big commotion as the Prime Minister of India was flying in, arriving from a foreign visit, so everything was put on hold and our flight and everyone else's was indefinitely delayed.

The backlog of passengers was such that every space in the airport was occupied, people sat on the floor, surrounded by bags and baggage, and they spread picnic cloths and settled in for a long wait. I went to enquire about our flight time; and by the time I came back, I found my Father-in-law lying on the floor with his head down, fast asleep. I thought: "He's realised the way to rest is to do what the locals do." We took the next flight to Jaipur; but by the time we got there, Dad felt unwell and was sick in the night. "This'll make you feel better." I said, drawing up a syringe full of anti-emetic. After twenty-four hours he was much better.

Amer, the old Jaipur Fort, was our next visit: perched high on an outcrop and mirrored in Maota Lake, the Fort's source of water. From the ramparts, one could see across the dry lands towards the Thar Desert. We sat in a *howrah* on an elephant's back to reach the Fort. The Maharaja of Jaipur had lived in the fort with his harem.

The next day we visited Hawa Mahal, the Palace of the Winds. The palace is so constructed as to catch and funnel breezes into all the many rooms. It looks like an ornate and beautiful red honeycomb. Air conditioning is not just a modern amenity.

We called on my niece, who entertained Dad with typical Rajasthani snacks. He found these difficult to eat so I suggested: "Take a bit of whatever is on offer and slip it in your pocket for the time being."

Back in Meerut at my parents' house, Dad met my father's cousin, Jagan Nath Arya. A professor of Sanskrit and Hindi, he had studied the origin of the most ancient of texts. His manners were charmingly old-fashioned, courteous, and kind and, like many academics, he was a man of very modest means. He described his extensive collection of books, including the ancient Vedic Texts, as his "jewels."

Dad and Jagan Arya often sought each other's company, as they were of a similar age. They exchanged ideas and discussed political and historical events. Jagan Arya always wore knee-length collarless tunics over tight trousers and a Gandhi Congress cap and read his texts through small wire-framed spectacles. He had an amazing memory and could recall the date, and even the hour, of historical events. The British Raj and the birth of Pakistan he could recall in detail, and he gave Dad the history of how we lost everything during the partition of India.

We left for Delhi again, on the final leg of our Indian Odyssey, and went back to Raj's place on Mall Road. My father-in-law is a convert to Catholicism, so I thought it would be a good idea to see the Catholic Cathedral in Delhi. We attended a Mass in the morning, which was spectacular. The Archbishop of Delhi, an impressive six-foot three inches tall, in his black and purple cassock, strode over to see us outside the Cathedral. He was very pleased to know of our relationship and invited us for tea at his Palace. I did not know you should kiss the Archbishop's ring, but Dad did – a sign of respect, he told me. We had tea in the Archbishop's garden and, after spending an hour, we left to visit the Mahatma Gandhi Memorial.

Gandhi's memorial in Raj Ghat is a simple area of white marble, surrounded by a wall covered with red and bright pink bougainvillea. Although hundreds of visitors were there, it seemed spacious and very peaceful.

To complete our visit, we toured Delhi by taxi for the whole day, taking in India Gate, Qutab Minar and Delhi Red Fort. The evening saw us at a performance of Dances of India, an amazing show giving an insight into the vastly different dances and cultures of the Indian sub-continent.

On the last day, I thought I would give my father-in-law an interesting gardening experience and I arranged to see the Presidential Garden. We were lucky that the President's Garden was open at the time and we were able to enjoy all the flora and fauna. We had a long talk with the Head Gardener, as my father-in-law was interested in all things botanic. We were also shown irrigation management for both drought and monsoon conditions. I did not know it was forbidden to take photographs, so we snapped away as much as we liked.

But now we were ready to return back home. The flight was 23.00 hours. We arrived at Palam Airport three hours early. The airport became fogbound after an hour and all flights were cancelled. The place became increasingly congested, every seat taken and then stranded passengers began to spread bedrolls out on any available floor space. No information came over the address system and the staff had no plan to resolve the situation.

This is India at its frustratingly patient best. I have been in England too long to take this philosophically, so I stormed over to the nearest desk and demanded what little information they knew.

"Excuse me," I bellowed, "I was booked on the cancelled 23.00 hours BA flight to Heathrow. It is now one o'clock in the morning and no announcements have been made. Does anyone here know what is happening? We've

169

been waiting two hours; nobody seems bothered to tell us all what the situation is!"

The staff behind the desk were calm and polite, but in no hurry to address my enquiry. They shook their sleepy heads. "We very much regret, sir, that we have no information as fog is outside our control."

"I suggest," I stormed, "that you ring your meteorological office and find out when the fog will clear!" I was due back at Barnsley Hospital the next day and I needed to know by how much we were likely to be delayed. After a few phone calls, they came back and said it would be sometime in the early morning.

I had left my father-in-law sitting on the floor beside our cases; but by the time I arrived back, he was fast asleep, with his head resting on a small suitcase. He had obviously been in India too long. There was no point in waking him. At 1.30am I again enquired, and they said: "All flights are cancelled until further notice." They had no arrangements for accommodation and no idea what to do with the thousands of stranded passengers within the terminal.

I shouted: "I know your efficiency will not extend to thinking what to do with thousands of passengers cluttering the departure hall. They're bedding down for the night, heating up tea on primus stoves. Are you equipped for a fire out there?" The staff looked taken aback. "Well," I added, "you'd better find accommodation for two passengers on the BA flight to Heathrow, *now!*"

By some miracle, they found a room in a five-star hotel. They even arranged a taxi to get us there. We dumped our luggage, flopped onto two luxurious double beds, and fell into an exhausted sleep. In the morning, we enjoyed a gigantic five-star breakfast.

We were going through the lobby when we came across a wedding in full swing. Dad was fascinated by all the paraphernalia. Women floated gracefully by in glittering saris of every colour. The bride wore the traditional red and gold. The men greeted each other loudly and strutted like peacocks in suits and turbans made of silk. Dad was carried off to join the ceremonies. He was conducted to a ringside seat near two red velvet thrones, where the bride and groom would sit. The thrones were beneath a richly decorated canopy. Also, under the canopy, a small fire burned, central to the ceremonies and blessings. We stayed at the wedding for an hour. The taxi called to return us to the airport.

We left the surreal, crazy world that is India and took the flight back to London without further incident.

21. Generations

SOMETIMES A SUCCESSFUL operation or treatment has effects that go well beyond a single generation.

Some years ago, Kate and I we were invited to a wedding. We had known the couple for many years. The reception was held in large marquees, tents, and barns on the groom's parents' farm. They had invited 400 guests, so it was a big occasion. There was a bar, a hog roast, a country dance band, a photographer, and a bouncy castle for the children.

Kate and I were standing in the field, watching the children play, when four beautiful young ladies strode purposefully towards us and stood two on each side of me. "Can we have our photograph taken with you?" they asked, then one of them chuckled: "*We* wouldn't be here if it wasn't for you!" That produced giggles amongst the girls and an amazed look from Kate.

"Have you got something to tell me, Sat?" Kate squared up to me, hands on hips. I was confused as I struggled to make sense of the situation. Out of the corner of my eye, I could see a man hurrying over the meadow towards us. "Hello, Mr Mehta, it's me, Colin. Do you remember me?"

"Of course, I remember you, Colin. How are you?"

Twenty-five years previously, Colin's accident was so serious that it nearly killed him. He had been using a carbide stone-cutting machine, when the cutting blade broke, and a large piece flew off at speed and sliced into his neck. It severed vital structures and he bled profusely. It all happened as I was just taking my gloves off, having finished my operating list. A nurse threw open the doors into the

172

operating theatre and panted: "Mr Mehta we *need* you in A&E! Guy's cut his neck, lost *a lot* of blood!"

I hurried down. The patient lay on a trolley, surrounded by the casualty officer and two nurses who were trying to stem the flow of blood that welled up relentlessly, spraying the curtains and making puddles on the floor. Blood pulsed and spurted from a huge gash in his neck. With my intimate knowledge of the anatomy of head and neck, I managed to find, in all that thick, red, pulsating mess, the severed carotid artery and jugular vein and clamped them with forceps. I called for the blood pump and pumped ten pints of blood into him as he lay in A&E and then transferred him up to the Emergency Theatre where we pumped him with a further six pints.

The narrow channel of the neck is crowded with vital blood vessels and nerves supplying the brain. Everything below the neck passes through this narrow junction to the head. Injury to the neck can cause paralysis or death. Wearing my magnifying operating spectacles, I carefully identified the carotid artery, the jugular vein and the severed muscles and sealed off the other bleeding points. The operation up to this point had taken five hours. We took a ten-minute break, during which time I came away from the table to stretch my legs. This would give time to see if we had caught all the bleeding points. The team and I returned to the table and proceeded with the final stages of the operation. I inserted a vacuum drain and closed the neck, muscle layers first then the skin. I sealed the wound with a spray and applied a thin layer of ribbon gauze. The operation had taken six hours. I saw him in Intensive Care Unit and at 1.30am I went home.

I went to see him the following morning. He was fully conscious and propped up on pillows. "How are you, Colin?" I enquired, "Well," he croaked "*I've got a bit of a*

173

sore throat!" I smiled and thought: how is that for Yorkshire Grit?

I knew that, as a nerve to the voice box had been severed, he would have a hoarse and husky voice forever. After two days in Intensive Care, Colin croaked: "I cannot lift my arm, Doctor, nor move my shoulder. Will I be able to play squash when I get out of here?" The nerves supplying the muscles of his shoulder had been cut and he would need physiotherapy in the future.

Later Colin showed me his very sore leg; and that remained a puzzle until I heard how, in haste to get Colin to the hospital, he had been bundled into the back of a van, and a tablecloth was wound round a car tyre and shoved into the hole in Colin's neck, then someone tried to slam the door shut, not realising that one of Colin's legs was sticking out of the van! In truth, this immediate action and the car tyre compression helped save Colin's life.

Colin had recounted the story of his near-death experience many times to his family. He must have spotted me across the field at the wedding and said: "Look girls, that's Mr Mehta over there. Remember? I told you he operated on me." And that is why the girls had come to thank me, because, in the fullness of time, Colin married and had produced his four beautiful daughters. We took photo after photo and had a happy reunion.

I will call this next patient Malcolm, though that was not his real name. He came to see me and gave a history of hoarseness of his voice, increasing over the previous six months. He was fit and healthy apart from the fact that he smoked cigarettes.

After investigations, examinations, X-Rays, and a biopsy, I diagnosed cancer of the vocal cords. We decided on an intensive course of radiotherapy lasting six months.

Malcolm's visits to the hospital were frequent, and during that time my Department got to know him well. He told us about his job as a gamekeeper in a beautiful local area. He maintained the buildings and controlled the birds, wild animals, and the herds of deer on the estate. He would bring a pheasant or a partridge to the Outpatient Clinic in a sealed box so that he could present it to the nurses or other staff as a "thank you" gift.

As the intensive radiotherapy treatment ended, it was clear he still had a residue of malignant growth left. A total removal of his voice box was the only course of action left to us. I explained that we needed to take a wide margin of muscles, cartilages and connecting blood vessels surrounding the previously irradiated and now shrunken cancerous tumour, in order to be sure we had removed the malignant area entirely.

Then the larynx is carefully dissected away from the rest of the airway connecting the mouth, nose, and food passage. I would then reconstruct the food passage, secure his windpipe back into the middle of his neck and insert a tracheostomy tube through which he would breathe. After that, I would repair the muscles and tissue I had cut away surrounding the tumour and close the wound.

As we discussed the operation, it became clear that the only thing Malcolm was concerned about was the fact that his shoulder muscles would be so weakened that he would not be able to bear the kick-back from the rifle he used every day in the course of his work as gamekeeper on the estate. But after careful consideration, Malcolm decided to have the operation.

We did it in Barnsley District General Hospital. He stayed for ten weeks in my ward, to make sure he could manage his new airway. During Malcolm's stay with us, I had inserted an artificial voice box and he learnt to speak again with the help of the Speech Therapist.

During our discussions Malcolm told me about his home life: "I was married but it didn't work out." He paused, drew breath, and continued in his croaky voice: "I've had four girlfriends as well." He cleared his throat and added: "Let's hope the one I'm with now is fifth time lucky!"

I asked: "And do you have any children, Malcolm?" He laughed and replied: "Thirty-two."

I quickly collected my thoughts. "Thirty-two children?"

"Yep," he grinned, "Some going, eh? At 64, I'm not doing so bad, am I?" He was a strong character with a good sense of humour, always cracking jokes and teasing the nurses. His girlfriend visited him most evenings and I saw her several times. Malcolm and his girl knew he would be on my ward for a considerable length of time. It became quite usual that, towards the end of visiting time, she would briefly pull the curtains round Malcolm's bed. One day I wanted to tell him about options available to restore his speech. I collected Ward Sister and we went onto the ward. The curtains round his bed were closed, so Sister pulled them aside and there was Malcolm and his girl in bed in what I shall call "a close embrace."

The surgery was a complete success: he was free of cancer and, with his lengthy recovery in hospital, he had learnt to cope well with his permanent tracheostomy tube and artificial voice box. He continued to attend the Combined ENT and Radiotherapy Clinic and usually brought something from the Estate as a gift for the nurses. After six months, he gave us the happy news that he was blessed with another child and we realised the baby must have been conceived while he was in my ward! On his next visit, he brought the new baby to the clinic to show us.

22. Our Family and Other Pets

THE STONE steps in our back garden lead down to a lower, paved area, where, tucked away underneath the weeping willow, is a small pond. In the pond are water lilies, irises and a good deal of duckweed. The aquatic wildlife consists of frogs, newts and very small fish.

A hedgehog once drowned in the pond, and we buried it with love and respect in a shoe box, underneath the apple tree. To prevent more hedgehog deaths, I hammered together a small wooden ladder, like a duckboard, and angled it against the edge of the pond, for future hedgehogs who mistake duckweed for *terra firma*, to paddle over to the steps and climb out. We had goldfish in the pond, but a heron came at six a.m. every morning for his breakfast, until all the fish were gone.

A small fountain plays merrily in the middle of the pond; and at one end, water gurgles and splashes from a height over stones and rocks. By early spring, the pond is covered with patches of frog spawn. I protect the spawn from our airborne visitor with a net stretched above the surface of the water, until I see the tiny frogs hop in and out of the borders.

As I said, the pond is situated under a willow tree, and leaves constantly drop into it; they then ferment into a putrid brew. So, every year, after the baby frogs have vacated the pond, I have to clean it. The newts I catch in a bucket; I clean the pond and then return them to their spring-cleaned home.

One sunny summer morning I decided to spring-clean the pond, looking forward to a slimy, stinking morning. I changed into an old tee-shirt and shorts, pulled on my full-length fishing wellingtons and, armed with three buckets and a wheelbarrow, I lowered myself into the watery black soup. I created a bridge across the pond from a wooden plank, upon which I could stand to haul myself out again. All was going well: I picked out the newts, transferred them to a small bucket, threw the remaining water and debris into the wheelbarrow and, when the wheelbarrow was full, hauled myself out onto my bridge and emptied the wheelbarrow onto the flower borders.

Eventually the plank became very slippery, and I slipped and fell headfirst into the pond.

I emerged covered in slime, duckweed and dead leaves, accompanied by the most pungently dirty smell. I wasn't injured so I got myself out of the pond and came to the side door of the house. There we have an outside tap and a hosepipe attached to it. As I was now dripping black slime wherever I walked, I decided to take all my clothes off outside the side door. It was quite a distance from the road, so I knew nobody could see me. When I was naked, I washed myself with a hosepipe and called Kate to tell her about the whole episode. But she did not hear me, so I decided to go inside without any clothes.

I did not know my wife was entertaining friends and neighbours to morning coffee in the kitchen, and she not only did not hear me, but she also did not see me as I walked from the utility room and headed upstairs to the shower. Our neighbours, however, watched in amazement as my bottom, with black and decomposing leaves sticking to it, ascended the stairs. Kate, still unaware of my dunking, tried to make out why our friends were suddenly all choking into their coffee cups.

Our gardener at that time was the father of six children, who had been made redundant from his previous job. He travelled ten miles on the bus to get to our house. I was very pleased with his gardening skills and his hard work.

He planted vegetables for us and his own family and gathered fruit in season from our orchard, but he was careful not to take too much. He constructed trellises, mended fences, gates and anything else that needed mending. He became a part of the family and so – when our eldest daughter Louise accidentally locked her bedroom door and then couldn't get it open again – he climbed up a ladder to her bedroom window and turned the key, resolving the situation. He comforted Louise and stepped over our son who was rolling about with laughter, on the upstairs landing floor. He taught our youngest daughter to count by slowly repeating the number of plants he was putting in the ground. He became invaluable.

The early eighties saw a fashion for brewing home beer and winemaking. Always an ardent follower of fashion, I decided to have a go. We have a good supply of apples, berries and other fruits in the garden. I decided to start with cider. Five demijohns and 20 bottles of cider, made from apples from our orchard, were slowly fermenting on the kitchen windowsill. Kate complained that the wonderful bubbling noises the fermentation produced made the kitchen sound like Frankenstein's laboratory and, furthermore, she said the jars *might explode*. I was given instructions to remove my fermentation jars from the kitchen.

I decided the warmer and sunnier greenhouse was a better place anyway. I stacked all five demijohns and the bottles on the workbench in the greenhouse. The extra warmth and sunshine boosted the fermentation considerably. A few hours later I went down to the greenhouse to check on my seedlings on the opposite side of the greenhouse to my demijohns and bottles. I lifted the covers on some early lettuce just sprouting through, when suddenly an enormous *Bang! Bang! Bang! Bang!* behind me, then a *Crack!* And the greenhouse roof caved in and sprinkled shards of glass on my head and everywhere else!

Luckily, the explosion was at my back. I turned to see the precious stuff, fruit of my labours, juice of our orchards, dripping from the workbench and running in rivulets onto the stone-flagged floor.

Kate heard the explosion and came running from the house. The greenhouse glass was completely blown. She combed slivers of glass from my hair for the next quarter of an hour. She muttered: "It's a good job you had your back turned, it could have been your eyes!" I did realise how silly I'd been, so she didn't need to keep rubbing it in. My cider ran uselessly down the flags and soaked into the soil. We both heaved a sigh of relief that the collateral damage was limited to new glass for the greenhouse and the end of my cider-making.

We had pets. Kate had Charlotte, her beloved Cairn terrier dog. Charlotte came to live with us very soon after we got married; she was a great companion for Kate when I was resident in the hospital over weekends, Friday to Monday, and on night duties. Charlotte was trained by Kate and we could take her anywhere without a lead, so closely did she follow Kate's heels. She was very playful and wonderful when the children came along. She lived to be fourteen, which in dog years is 98. She is buried in a quiet spot in the garden, underneath the chestnut trees.

Kate also kept five Rhode Island Red hens. They roamed loose in the orchard by day but were kept safe from foxes in a hen coop by night. Kate looked after them exceptionally well, but on those rare occasions when it was after dusk before she got around to gathering them into the coop, they roosted in the apple, pear and plum trees. As a result, they first had to be found and dislodged from the branches; then, flapping and protesting, they were put to bed

180

in the hen coop. They were prolific in their egg-laying, so we ate lots of sponge cake.

We encouraged our children to have a pet of their own choosing; to be organised enough to clean and look after it, to care for it and understand its various needs; to be kind to the animals and to understand when they die, how to mourn and bury them, and eventually to move on and maybe get another pet.

Our eldest daughter Louise had two cats, two rabbits and a guinea pig. The cats were hyperactive toms and flew, claws out, to cling onto the best sitting room curtains. They dined on choice pieces of chicken breast from our daughter's plate and I'm sure they slept in her bed, although that was forbidden. The rabbits had a lovely hutch and a run, which she moved daily to fresh grass in the orchard. She often carried them up to her bedroom, where they loped gently around the room whilst she did her homework.

One of the rabbits got loose and ate all our neighbours' rose bushes. Louise had to spend her pocket money on a tray of replacement rose bushes. She called, tray in hand, with an abject apology written on her best Pierrot notelet paper.

Paul could not be bothered with pets, but he *did* have a fish tank in his room and managed to keep a goldfish for a while. We enrolled him in the Royal Society for the Protection of Birds, but sport was really what took Paul's interest.

As I've already mentioned, Ollie and Pepe, the budgerigars, lived in Clare's room. We always knocked before entering, as a frenzy of startled feathers and a squawk from the top of the curtains alerted us to the fact that they were on the loose. Clare also had a mallard drake and duck named Donald and Daisy. They came to live with us as chicks with their foster- mother, Milly, the hen.

Milly, who belonged to our youngest daughter Jane, proved to be a most attentive mother to Donald and Daisy. Milly loved to sit on Jane's lap, eyeing the world with that sideways look that hens have, and enjoying Jane's gentle stroking of her soft brown feathers. Jane even entered her in the school pet competition; but, as there was no-one else with a pet hen, they were in a class of their own and there was no medal for them.

It was the responsibility of Clare and Jane to collect the eggs from the garden for the kitchen. Clare's egg collecting mishap described earlier is etched on her memory, leaving her seriously traumatised for life, no doubt.

We also had six huge white Aylesbury ducks. I brought them as large fluffy ducklings from a farmhouse in South Yorkshire. We settled them down in the bottom shed for the night. To our dismay, in the morning they could not stand up, they had lost the strength in their legs and lay on their backs with their legs in the air. We did not know what to do so we asked our next-door neighbour, a vet, but he could give no answer.

Kate decided to go and ask the Farm Shop where she bought all the pet food. They concluded that the ducklings had been used to feed containing growth hormone. Kate bought some hormone laced feed and by the following morning they were back on their feet. We opened the shed door and out they tumbled, running all over the garden, their recovery complete.

These ducklings became very large ducks, but we weaned them off the hormones. They laid eggs all over the garden, under bushes, on the shed roof and in the dog's bowl: strange places, so we never ate them.

We invited children passing by in the lane on their way home from school to come in and see the animals. The only rule was that they be sure to shut the gate. During autumn, they knew they could also collect conkers from the ground.

As an experiment, I thought it a good idea to have a nanny goat. I asked one of my farmer friends to loan me a goat. We drove a stake into the orchard grass and tethered the imaginatively named Nanny to it. We milked the goat twice a day, a time-consuming task, as it took one to hold her and the other to do the milking. "Ah! Before you go, you'll have to help me milk Nanny," Kate often said as I was about to leave for the hospital. No matter what the weather, bucket in hand, off we went, to milk Nanny. Our neighbour, out walking his dog often stopped by to sing *"The Hills are alive with the Sound of Music"*

Even tethered, Nanny ate everything in the orchard including the bark of the trees, the raspberry canes, the gooseberry bushes and the top of the compost heap. It was great fun to start with; but gradually, as our farmer friend knew, we found looking after her and milking twice a day quite onerous. The children did not like salty goat's milk, even when disguised with Ovaltine. In the end, we decided we should let the goat go and returned Nanny to the farm.

As the ducks became bigger, we made a large pen for them. The guinea pigs lived in a smaller adjoining pen. When we fed the ducks, the guinea pigs would nip through the little gate, steal some duck food, then run back through the gate, to their own pen. The cereal we fed attracted big rats to the garden. We called in the Council's Vermin Department. The Officer remarked: "You've got some very healthy rats, lovely glossy coats, they've got." He continued: "What with the duck eggs and the cereal, they run along here," he indicated a straight pathway, "to the pond for a drink. What more could a rat want?" He promised to visit us regularly until every last rat was gone, and he was as good as his word.

Because of the rats, we decided the Aylesbury ducks should go too. We explained to the children that the ducks were going on holiday. I arranged for the local Travelling People to call, but asked them to pick the ducks up in a sensitive way. They caught them by the legs, and took them upside down, squawking and flapping, to the van on the front drive. Louise was outraged by the sight of her beloved white monsters in such distress.

By this time, we had two more children so decided to have some home help. Fortunately, one of my ward staff's sisters was available. The lady had been home help in a number of houses and was conversant with the work. She was truly wonderful and a great help to Kate. She would answer the phone with a polite "Mr Mehta's Residence, may I help you?"

She was with us for ten years. After that, we had another help who managed to put up with us for twenty years. She suited us well and soon became part of the family. She had been trained as a cook by the Royal Navy. As a Wren she had served in Portsmouth, then married a man in the army and they were posted to Malaysia. She had two grown daughters and a son.

She had a gift for making order out of chaos. This wonder of military organisation swept all before her, into a large tidy pile, destined for the dustbin. Kate only had to breathe her name to send the children into paroxysms of tidying, momentarily of course.

Louise would dash upstairs to hide love letters, take half eaten cake out of her knicker drawer or extract pizza from underneath her bed. Paul swept books and papers off the floor and stuffed them into his overfilled cupboard, until one day, the cupboard could hold no more, and the door came off its hinges. Clare flashed about with a dustpan and

184

brush underneath the birdcage in her bedroom. Jane, tidy even to Royal Navy standards, simply smoothed over her bedcover and counted the folded socks in her underwear drawer. All was ship-shape and Bristol Fashion on one day a week in our house.

On the occasions that we opened our garden to the Senior Citizens in a nearby Residential Home, or the Hospice Day Patients, our home help was a total treasure. She would have none of your shop-bought scones and cakes but insisted on baking them herself. She was in her element when catering to a large crowd. She filled Kate's many tea pots with speed and skill. To her eternal credit, she taught me to make scones for our hospice visitors, which I could make fresh on the day.

Bonfire Night was a particular favourite of hers. We held it in the orchard, at the farthest point from the house, and we set up a field kitchen. It was a bank of steaming hot *bain marie* dishes, a hostess trolley and a barbecue; flood lit and sheltered as it was, under a large awning near the old apple tree. Here she was "In Charge" and the feeding of the five thousand ran as smoothly as it did in Jesus's time. We served baked potatoes with baked beans, chicken curry and rice, hot crispy garlic bread, parkin cake and bonfire toffee and drank hot mulled wine.

23. Relatives

AS I'VE ALREADY MENTIONED, the first time I met Kate's paternal grandma, 'Mopsy,' was at my wedding. I was very honoured and impressed that she made a special effort to attend her granddaughter's wedding. She came with her daughter Jeanne and Kate's cousins. Mopsy was a regal figure beneath her hat with the large white ostrich feather wound around the crown. Mopsy only had one hat, and the feather went on the hat for weddings and was removed for funerals. She carried a cream-coloured Pekingese in her arms.

We saw Mopsy again when Kate and I and our new baby daughter Louise visited her at Aunt Jeanne's beautiful rambling old Rectory in Warwickshire. Mopsy had a comfortable and spacious ground floor flat there. She chuckled: "It's great we have some new blood in the family." She brought a large atlas from her bookcase and we located my birthplace. She asked about my family background and my upbringing in India.

She was a Huguenot whose aristocratic ancestors fled to England during the French Revolution to escape the guillotine. "My father was a tea merchant in Imperial China, before the cultural revolution," she said, "I did not see much of him and, as my mother was dead, I was brought up by my married sister." Mopsy's room was filled with Chinese artefacts and antiques.

Kate's grandfather Eric had married Mopsy after he graduated from Durham University with first class honours in Latin, Greek and Theology. He was ordained into the Church of England. As he was a minister, they moved, with their growing family, from place to place.

The Reverend Eric was offered a Deanship at St

George's Chapel, Windsor Castle. He turned it down saying: " I want to serve ordinary people. A simple faith is the best."

And that is exactly what he did. His Rectory was the hub of the town or village, and he and Mopsy became the community's benefactors, counsellors and aid wherever they were posted. He once said, with a wry smile: "I conduct many *quiet* weddings, followed very shortly afterwards by *large* christenings!'

In the days before the NHS, there was an outbreak of both measles and scarlet fever in their village. Isolation between family members was impossible in the small cottages, so the Rectory became a makeshift hospital, with measles beds on one side of the house and scarlet fever beds on the other. Mopsy was the Nurse. Town and village meetings were held in the Rectory; the Tennis Club, the WI meetings, the Bridge Club and many more organisations operated out of the Rectory.

During the Second World War the American Airforce was billeted in the Rectory, and Eric and Mopsy moved to a nearby cottage. GIs staying in the Rectory said: "Say, Ma'am, we don't feel right callin' ya the Rector's wife, hope you like Mopsy, cause that's what we'd like to call ya." Mopsy liked the proposal and the name stuck.

During the War, their eldest son was in the Docklands, fighting fires and digging victims from blitzed East London. Their second son was a 23-year-old Padre to the Forces, sent to the front line. Their fourth son, aged 19, my father-in -law, was a radio operator in the skies over the Middle East.

Their third son was a Squadron Leader in Bomber Command's Elite Pathfinders 7 and 8 Squadrons. He and his squadron undertook many night-time sorties into the heart of Nazi territory, but in November 1943 he was shot down and killed over Germany. Kate and I never met Hugh, but we and

187

our family are so personally grateful for his skill, courage and bravery. He had flown at least 37 successful operational sorties when he was killed.

An extract from the Aircrew notice board page 167 – Sqdn. Ldr. Eric Hugh Montgomery Nesbitt 7 Squadron – gives the following: Squadron leader Nesbitt took off from RAF Oakington, Cambridge, at 16.56 in the afternoon of November 1943 and his destination was Berlin, lying deep in the heart of Germany. It was known as the Big City by its crews and heavily defended by night fighters and anti-aircraft guns. The Pathfinders were first over the target where the coloured flares they dropped would mark the points for the following Bomber stream. Either on the way to Berlin or on the way back, the Lancaster crashed at Hope, near Hannover. There were no survivors.

During peacetime Mopsy was involved in voluntary and social work. She was very active on the panel of The League of Friends of Oswestry hospital. She organised fundraising events for many good causes in the days before the Welfare State and had, what she called 'Open House' for one and all. Rector Eric had ministries in Durham, Shropshire and Lincolnshire. His heart, however, was always in the Welsh valleys where he was born and where he is now laid to rest.

A while ago, Kate received a telephone call, "Hello" said the voice, "My name is Peter, I'm your distant cousin!"

Kate was astounded, but even more so when he said: "I'm going to Germany to visit your uncle Hugh's war grave, would you like to come with me?" They talked for a while, but she gave a non-committal answer. A short while later, Peter phoned back clarifying that he *was* eighty years old and furthermore, his wife Angela would be travelling to Germany too.

I said "Go! It's a great opportunity for you to honour the brave uncle you never knew!" Kate is very grateful to those who fought for our nation's freedom. She plants a commemorative poppy near the pond in our garden every year on November 11th and has done for the last forty-three years. "I'd *love* to come!" Kate said, and they made arrangements to meet on Dover Railway station. "You'll know it's me by my bright red sweater," said Peter; Kate replied: "OK. I'll be wearing a big red rose in the lapel of my coat."

Peter and Angela had contacted The War Graves Commission for directions to the exact location of the grave. They took turns at the wheel of their car and drove Kate through France and Germany.

Hanover War Cemetery, near Seelze, is where beneath headstone No 6A8. lie the ashes of Squadron Leader Eric Hugh Montgomery Nesbitt. His crew are laid to rest on either side of him. They were returning from a raid on Berlin, during which, amongst the buildings they destroyed were: the Kaiser Wilhelm Memorial Church, Charlottenburg Castle, the Berlin Zoo, the British, French, Italian and Japanese Embassies, Siemen's Electrical Group Factory, the Alkett Tank Works, the Ministry of Weapons and Munitions, the Waffen SS Administrative College and the barracks of the Imperial Guard at Spandau.

We will be forever grateful that Peter and Angela contacted us. Kate found their company delightful, they got on famously. "There's a Christmas Market in Hamelin, how about we go tomorrow?" Said Peter and they did.

We determined our newly discovered family members come to visit us at home. "You are *never* going to motor all the way from Hampshire to Edinburgh to see your son, you *must* stay overnight with us, we are halfway," we said, and so it was that the splendid Peter and Angela came to stay. The conversation over dinner sparkled with Peter's *own* adventures as a pilot in the RAF. "I flew most aircraft of the day, from Spitfires to Vampire Jets."

Angela said: "Yes, he's taken planes to Venice, Suez Canal, Cyprus, Khartoum, Asmara, Somalia, Baghdad and Kanpur. I think he's a nomad really, but that suits me too."

Peter and Angela's worldwide travels by land, sea and air are well documented, and in the words of his lovely granddaughter," There isn't a beach in the *world* that they haven't rocked up on, including the Galapagos Islands!"

24. Lull Before the Storm

DURING THE LONG summer recesses that universities have, Sheffield University would use its facilities to host courses open to the public. We even had the option of weekly boarding in the students' residences. The Mehta family decided to enrol, all six of us, and stay in the student accommodation at night. Louise split her day and had tennis coaching in the morning and belly danced all afternoon. Paul went for tennis all day and Clare and Jane joined the children's adventure group.

Hot air ballooning appealed to both Kate and me and our long dreamed of flights of fancy became real. Two expert balloonists from Bristol strode into the classroom bearing a collection of maps, two-way radios and a short film. We studied the weather, the clouds, the wind direction and the weather forecast for the next few hours. We spread maps on the desks and pored over Ordnance Survey, Air Corridor and *Angry Farmers* maps.

The Ordnance Survey map of the area gave us the land below; we took particular note of electricity pylons. The Air Corridor mapped out the pathways that aircraft, large and small, would take. The final *Angry Farmers* map is relevant to Hot Air Balloonists, as the loud Whoosh! of the burners that keep the balloon aloft disturbs farming livestock in the field beneath. To gain height and silently drift over a field without causing a stampede, a "cow burner" is employed: it gives a silent boost to the heat, up we rise, and, unbeknown to the livestock beneath, we silently glide by.

That evening, we gathered on a large grassy field near the university to view our unique and beautiful transport. It comprised a huge red and yellow striped balloon known as the envelope; various ropes; a wicker basket; and a gas cylinder. Under instruction, we lit the burner and with a *whoosh*, we directed the flame into the envelope until, inflated with hot air, it rose majestically from the ground. Then we let it down again. There ended our first lesson.

The following day, an early morning mist hung over the field, and as dawn was breaking, we gathered for our first flight. The expert pilots, wearing bright orange boiler suits, directed us as we inflated the balloon envelope slowly over a period of an hour.

Gradually the hot air caused the envelope to rise up and some of us held onto the wicker basket whilst the rest climbed in and cast off. We rose slowly from the field, the mist had lifted and in the morning sun, we drifted towards the city of Sheffield. The balloon was now about 2,500 feet over the outskirts of the city. Suburban sprawl and neat housing estates lay below, shining in the morning light. The sky above was cloudless and blue. In the houses beneath, the people of Sheffield were waking up to a new day.

"Halloo!" early risers called up from their gardens, breakfast bowls in their hands, "Hey! Down here!" They waved, we waved back and sailed on. As we were travelling at the same speed and in the same direction as the wind, it did not whistle past us, we could neither feel nor hear it. It was very peaceful. The burner gave us control over the height, but the direction is entirely in the hands of the flow of air – we were just blown along like thistledown. "Now you know why we study the weather so carefully before we set off!" said David, our instructor and pilot, "No flying over the M1 motorway, no flying near Doncaster/Sheffield Airport, no flying over Tinsley Cooling Towers etc etc." He grinned. And so, we glided on and on; it was wonderful.

Eventually our time in the basket was up and it was time to give others a go. David pulled a rope, opening the balloon on the top. The balloon descended and we landed at a bus stop on a housing estate!

The few people who were about pretended we were not there, nothing unusual was going on. As I've said, the English gift for understatement never ceases to amaze me, but to ignore a thirty-foot red and yellow hot air balloon landing at a bus stop at eight o'clock on a Sunday morning is taking "Keep Calm and Carry On" a bit far. The only being that saw anything unusual was a furiously barking dog, straining at the leash. "Stop that, Trigger. You silly boy!" his owner yelled, and she walked on by.

A group of Punk Rockers, probably on their way home from a party, crossed the road to investigate, maybe we might be from outer space, maybe Sheffield City Transport might have new vehicles; anything is feasible on the way home from an all-night party. We enlisted their help to hang onto the sides of the wicker basket whilst we clambered out. The Punk Rockers hung onto the basket with great gusto and strength; they even gleefully held us fast to the pavement as a Panda Car pulled up and two members of South Yorkshire Police strolled over. The police pointed out that we were causing an obstruction, and could we please get airborne and move on?

Kate was in another balloon. She was travelling higher and in a different direction, out over the fields and countryside beyond Sheffield, towards Penistone. We in the first balloon were present to greet them and I was able to video Kate's landing. The balloon descended smoothly but the basket hit the side of a hedge and Kate and crew landed upside down in a corn-stubble field. Thrown out of the basket – but all was well! Kate enjoyed the rough and tumble of ballooning and all she suffered were some bruising and corn stubble scratches.

The ballooning course was so interesting that a number of us wanted to buy a balloon as a group hobby. It never came to anything but was a great thought. We got to know everyone fairly well, as not only did we spend whole days together up in a wicker basket, but evenings as well in the bar and having a meal together.

On the final evening, a celebratory dinner was held, after which entertainment was provided by the Belly Dancing group. I produced a short film of our ballooning and sent a video copy to all the members on our course.

I've already mentioned our parish church has a unique charity known as The Suzy Fund, begun by Brian and his family. One of my contributions to the fund was to hold an annual Plant Sale, together with Derek, a likeminded friend, either in his garden or mine. In those days, garden centres had yet to become big business and the horticultural establishments that existed at the time could not compete with *our* prices. We got most of our plants from green-fingered friends, growing in egg boxes, plastic yoghurt pots and any other disposable containers. The Plant Sale grew – you could even say it mushroomed – both in size and diversity as we became more ambitious. We even had our own horticultural expert, Dennis.

Dennis had gained a degree from Askham-Byram Horticultural College and was a regular exhibiter at Chelsea Flower Show. He had a special interest in hanging baskets and could get plants from nurseries on a sale-or-return basis. He acquired a great selection of bedding plants and herbs for us, and he brought his famous baskets. We could also boast amongst our stall holders Graham, an expert on fuchsias, but the rest of us had acquired our knowledge in a more haphazard way.

I like to think our customers enjoyed the amateur status of our enterprise and were tolerant of the odd drooping leaf, greenfly or slug. One year however, we had a complaint from one of our most valued customers. The previous year she had bought all our best quality trailing petunias for hanging baskets outside her front door. But this year she complained loudly about our happy-go-lucky plant labelling.

To be fair to anyone but Dennis, the leaves of petunias and cucumbers *are* very similar. However, our customer was not amused. She thundered that hers was the only house on the street that had a bumper crop of cucumbers hanging over the front porch. We took immediate action: we ushered her over to sit in Dennis's seat, whilst we hurried over to the refreshment tent for a glass of wine and a plate of cheese nibbles. We also boxed up a selection of our finest plants, accurately labelled, and it all ended happily.

Unpredictable weather was another hazard and prompted endless discussion as we speculatively eyed the skies for tell-tale signs, racked our brains for weather folklore and took note of the meteorological forecasts. On one occasion, the day prior to the Plant Sale, we had just finished laying out 180 trays of pre-ordered plants, all over the back lawn, down the path and under the trees in the orchard, when we heard the weather forecast of impending frost coming our way that very night, with minus temperatures and clear skies.

Kate and I set to work raiding the dustbin for newspapers, hunting the house for tablecloths and clearing the airing cupboard of bedsheets; and, in the gathering dusk, we covered half an acre of tender bedding plants with our makeshift protection.

Kate had gone inside to make dinner when I noticed only one item remained uncovered: an expensive bought-in standard acer tree. What to do? How to cover it? I hit on a brilliant idea. Kate's old dance dress, hanging in the wardrobe, would be perfect: so I covered the tree with the full-length ball gown. The following morning dawned crisp and clear, the frost covered everything in a stiff and sparkling coat. As we reached the end of the lawn, Kate stopped when she spotted my clever tree cover.

"Aaaggh!" she shrieked, "What is that? Is that *my dance dress?*" I now know there is no such thing as an *old* dance dress. Breakfast was in silence that morning.

I remember singing *"Our God Reigns"* and He obliged with a deluge of Biblical proportions.

Dennis had a regular stand at Chelsea Flower Show and one year he invited Kate and me to accompany him. We were to help him in setting up his stand the day prior to public admission. Pinning on our *Exhibitors* badges, we set to work setting out Dennis's stall. "Thanks, that's looking great," said Dennis, "why don't you two go and have a wander round?" It was a golden opportunity to visit the whole show before the crowds that would come on the following day.

"The Queen's coming this afternoon," I smiled, "and the press." Kate was impressed. "And a few celebs," I added, "and us."

"Yes, and all for the price of helping Dennis set up his stall!" enthused Kate.

We admired towering displays of perfect blooms, we took notes on garden design, and we chatted with renowned experts on everything from rare orchids to compost heaps, as we mingled with TV celebrities of the gardening world. We met Geoff Smith, Alan Titchmarsh, Joanna Lumley, Jerry Hall and Gary Sobers. Dennis came along to share a glass of champagne with us and fellow exhibitors.

We watched a broadcasting crew with their sound booms and cameras make a commentary for BBC evening news. We became aware of a number of people gathered around the rose exhibits; the entourage then parted to reveal John Major, the Prime Minister!

Ever since I was able to buy my first box Brownie, I have been a keen photographer and I had my enormous video camera perched on my shoulder. Back then, video cameras were industrial-sized. Out of curiosity, I went across and videoed not only the roses but also the Prime Minister's group. The Prime Minister smiled into my camera and enquired of me: "Got all the pictures you need? I'll move on, if that's OK." He must have thought I was from TV India!

We knew the Queen would visit the Chelsea Show and, to our delight, in the late afternoon sunshine, the Queen and Royal Family surrounded Dennis's exhibit and admired his stand.

The day proved inspirational, as later that year we decided to improve our own garden. Kate and I decided to build an herb garden – incorporating several different areas. We planted the herbs on three of our vegetable areas and had over a hundred and fifty varieties, including fifty medicinal herbs. We planted culinary herbs, perfumed herbs, dye-giving herbs, insect-repellent herbs and cleansing and disinfectant herbs. The Physic Garden of medicinal herbs we researched particularly well because no self-respecting medieval doctor would be without his Physic Garden: witch hazel, bladderwort, digitalis, evening primrose, rue, echinacea, ladies' mantle, gingko biloba and many more we planted and labelled. We even produced a stylish pamphlet, printed in Gothic print, on how the herbs in our Physic Garden would have been used long ago.

For several years in the spring, we enlisted friends to help put up two huge marquees on the lawn. They stayed up all summer and we entertained senior citizens from nearby residential homes and patients and staff from our local hospice day centres. The visitors, on warm summer days, meandered along the winding paths, pausing every now and then to sit and inhale the perfumes from the aromatic herbs and flowers, hear the bees humming and the dragonflies skimming the pond. For a while, our visitors could forget their pain and frailty and step back into a green oasis of tranquillity.

The bottom of the garden held a hidden delight as they passed under the arches, thick with fragrant flowering jasmine, through the wicket gates and into the dappled-shaded orchard. At the far end of the orchard, spread like a vast green cathedral, there rose to the sky the branches of tall chestnut and sycamore trees. Then it was back to the top lawn for tea and scones under the marquee and a bit of gentle conversation.

We served home-made cream teas and cake, and for the nurses fresh fruit, as they always seemed to be on a diet. On several occasions a neighbour demonstrated her Tai Chi, and another neighbour, known as The Singing Doctor, came to sing. We had a shower of rain once, so we all went into the house and got out our guitars and one of the hospice carers did a turn.

One such day, our decorator, whose hobby is bodybuilding, was busy painting our sitting room walls. Kate mentioned that one of our wheelchair-bound guests had never been as far as the orchard, as none of us was strong enough to get her there. He asked for the afternoon off, went home to change his clothes and came back to push that wheelchair; so, the guest in question had a lovely young man with a Charles Atlas body to push her wheelchair to the orchard and around the garden for the rest of the day. As our guests got back onto the minibus, we presented every lady with a small posy of fragrant flowers, and to the nurses we gave pot plants.

"I've done a silly thing!" said Kate as she put down the phone one day. "I've asked *Yorkshire Life* magazine if they'd like to feature our garden!"

"Mmmm?" I said absentmindedly, and I continued to read the newspaper.

"Yes," Kate went on, "They said: 'Ah! You need to speak to our gardening *expert*. Hold on a minute, I'll put you through." I sat up and took notice.

So a date was arranged and, in the days and weeks before *Yorkshire Life's* gardening expert's visit, we gardened by day and night. We literally combed the lawns to green perfection; plastic plant labels were replaced with wooden home-made labels, and even the house brick that held the greenhouse door closed was painted green by Kate "to blend in a bit and look as if it's *not* a brick."

So it was that *Yorkshire Life's* gardening feature writer and expert photographer came to tea. The article she wrote was aptly entitled: *The Couple Who Knew Nothing about Gardening.*

On the first Saturday in November, the action moved to the orchard, where our bonfire glowed and our garden lights illuminated our field-kitchen, serving hot food. The field kitchen was the domain of Pam, our treasured home help. The fireworks, set off to music, were spectacular as they rose into the night sky; and to me, this is not Guy Fawkes Night but Diwali, the Indian Festival of Light. We invited friends and neighbours, although our immediate neighbours needed no invitation – they just came over to help as soon as they saw the bonfire glow. We raised funds for the Suzy Fund in this way.

A friend suggested I part-share in buying a gymnasium with him. He later sold the property as a going concern but kept the profit from the sale. However, he did send to our house a heavy commercial sunbed and the tokens to operate it, as my share of the sale. Kate was very annoyed and refused to have it in the house, so I suggested she could sun herself in the garage.

"Certainly not!" she shrieked, "I'm lying there, and the gardener loses his eyesight when he comes to get the lawnmower!"

Trays of my geraniums had the sun ray treatment in a bid to bring them on, but all to no avail. Eventually the sunbed went to the rubbish tip. Here we were, enjoying the pleasures of our life, little knowing what was round the corner...

Epilogue

MY HEART operation affected me emotionally, and for two years I knew my body had been cured – but my mind had suffered a battering.

Immediately after the operation I walked with Kate every day, making a pub at the end of it, our goal. The distance between pubs increased and gradually I became more and more fit. It took me three months to get back to normal walking and I did not go back to work in the hospital for six months.

After the operation I felt depressed and wanted to get back to my work and gardening. Our close friends Brian and Lynne, the couple who began The Suzy Fund, suggested I spend a week in retreat at Mount St Bernard Abbey. We thought that would be helpful in coming to terms and accepting the situation.

Brian is a close family friend and early in his life he wanted to be a priest. But after living two years in a seminary, he decided it was not his calling. To cope with the turmoil in his life, he spent time in the Abbey in Leicestershire.

His mentor and confidant at the Abbey, Brother Thomas, was still there, so Kate booked a week's stay for me. Kate's wonderful cousin, also named Brian, drove me to the Abbey; and, after afternoon tea, they left me there.

There were seven services in the chapel over the twenty-four-hour day. Brother Thomas said that, on account of my delicate health, I could miss the 3am first service of the day. I joined in the many discussion groups, spent time in the large library, walked in the grounds and helped to collect vegetables from the garden and pick fruit from the orchard. The doors were locked at 7pm. Brother Thomas

201

arranged to meet me after supper and go for a walk in the garden, discussing my recuperation and how to cope with what had happened. He had great depth of knowledge and has been a great help to me ever since. Apart from that, we discussed football and his early childhood and how he became a Brother in the Abbey. We often finished with a tipple of whisky.

Because of the drugs I now take daily, my skin is sensitive and itchy. My clothing must be loose, and I cannot wear a belt to hold my trousers up, nor can I have elastic in my underpants, they must have a drawstring waist. Due to the high alert at airports now, I must surrender my braces to the plastic tray and try and make it through the body scanner without causing a sensation. I warn the security staff, but they take my braces anyway. On one occasion my trousers dropped to the floor, to the amusement of airport security staff and passengers. In addition, the wires used to close my breastbone in my chest give interesting noises when I go through the airport body scan, and so I find myself once again of special interest to the security staff.

I had gradually started recuperating with a little light gardening. Luckily, the year of the operation was warm and sunny, the garden flourished and grew in abundance. I had a regular help in the garden, and he banned me from digging or lifting anything heavy.

We had a barbecue most days that summer, and I was so thankful that I was alive to watch the family enjoying a meal in the sunshine.

One day we harvested beetroot and salad and we had a lunchtime family barbecue. In the evening I went to the bathroom and was very upset to see red residue in the toilet. Immediately I thought that there was blood in the stool. I thought it could be due to the aspirin I was taking for thinning the blood, following the operation. I discussed the situation with Kate, and we decided I should contact my colleague in General Surgery.

He was very kind and suggested I undergo a colonoscopy (an examination using a camera) the following day. I took a suspension of powder that is the medical equivalent of a scouring pad for the gut. But that evening I remembered the quantity of beetroot salad I had with my lunchtime barbecue.

I rang my colleague, but he was having none of it. "I've arranged it, Sat. I'll look forward to seeing you tomorrow." The industrial strength laxative kept me awake all night and the revelation from the colonoscopy was – as we all knew by then – an overdose of beetroot!

Afterword

MY FIRST BOOK *Flying with a Broken Wing* is about my childhood at the time of the Partition in India. My family were Hindu landowners; but when I was five years old, my world fell apart when the British left India and Pakistan was created.

Overnight, on 14th August 1947, our family and farmlands found themselves in Pakistan. We had to leave our ancestral home and so we became destitute refugees.

We spent a few months in refugee camps. Then we moved to a one-roomed slum in Meerut. When not in school, my time was spent on the street. Homework was done in the park under the shady trees, as home was too small and hot. A dog bite, a near-drowning, leaping across rooftops, riverside cremations, and marijuana cakes: I have a personal story involving each one. Times were hard; but, because we saw with the eyes of children, we felt no fear for the future and had no interest in the past.

As I've already mentioned in this book, I broke my arm when I was a boy. The wound refused to heal and amputation was imminent. As the purchase of an artificial arm was beyond my parents' means, I would spend my life handicapped. But by sheer chance, Robert Roaf, a Liverpool bone surgeon of world renown, visited India to teach new techniques for the most severe of bone conditions; and I got a second chance. The gratitude I felt for the great man's skill and expertise shaped the rest of my life.

I won a scholarship to one of only five universities in the whole of the Indian subcontinent to study Medicine. To pay for this, I tutored maths during my holidays. So, fully qualified and with skills in medicine, surgery, and obstetrics, I was ready for the world. I left for England in 1966, when

204

the country was at fever pitch as the football World Cup was in full swing. I had never seen a television – and the television in the doctors' residence was perpetually tuned to football.

Readers will know from a previous chapter that in England I visited my hero, Professor Roaf, to say a big personal *Thank You*.

This new book has been the story of my life in England. My professional life has been interesting and rewarding. My family and social life is wonderful. I have taken the country to my heart and they have adopted me.

In 1970 I married Kate and we are blessed with four beautiful children and five granddaughters. Now I have time to reflect and look back down the long road I have travelled. I realise the extraordinary events that have shaped my life.

After fifty years in Britain, I have written this book to give insight into the life of a surgeon and a family man, settled in a country which embraced me and gave me the privilege to serve its people.

The heroes of this book are you, my readers; also, my family, my friends, my patients and professional colleagues. *You* are my inspiration. My heartfelt thanks to you!

Also in Nettle Books

Flying with a Broken Wing
Sat Mehta

Flying with a Broken Wing tells the true story of a boy
growing up in India in turbulent times. Sat Mehta was
five years old when he and his family became refugees,
caught up in the biggest migration in modern history at
the time of Independence. His home was destroyed, his
uncle murdered. The Mehtas became destitute. Later,
Sat suffered a broken arm – complications set in and
amputation seemed inevitable. But world-famous
surgeon Robert Roaf gave Sat a second chance. The
gratitude Sat felt for the great man's skill shaped the rest
of his life. He qualified as a doctor and arrived in
England, where he has lived and worked for 30 years.
ISBN: 978-0-9561513-2-2   **£10**

www.ingramcontent.com/pod-product-compliance
Lightning Source LLC
Chambersburg PA
CBHW051958090426
42741CB00008B/1452